JUST THE RULES!

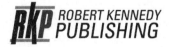

ROBERT KENNEDY
PUBLISHING

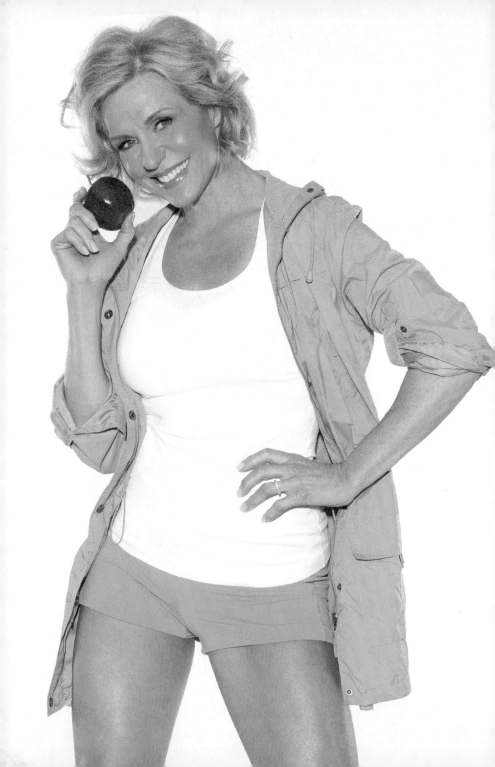

JUST THE RULES!

Tosca's Guide to Eating Right

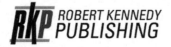
ROBERT KENNEDY PUBLISHING

Published by Robert Kennedy Publishing
400 Matheson Blvd. West, Mississauga, ON
L5R 3M1 Canada
Visit us at **www.eatcleandiet.com,
www.rkpubs.com** and **www.toscareno.com**

Library and Archives Canada Cataloguing
in Publication

Reno, Tosca, 1959-
    The eat-clean diet presents--
    just the rules: Tosca's guide to
    eating right / Tosca Reno.

ISBN 978-1-55210-093-6
1. Nutrition. 2. Food habits. I. Title.
RA784.R46 2011   613.2   C2011-900671-5

10 9 8 7 6 5 4 3 2 1

Distributed in Canada by
NBN (National Book Network)
67 Mowat Avenue, Suite 241
Toronto, ON
M6K 3E3

Distributed in USA by
NBN (National Book Network)
15200 NBN Way
Blue Ridge Summit, PA
17214

Printed in Canada

Robert Kennedy Publishing
BOOK DEPARTMENT

MANAGING DIRECTOR **Wendy Morley**	ART DIRECTOR **Gabriella Caruso Marques**
SENIOR EDITOR **Amy Land**	ASSISTANT ART DIRECTOR **Jessica Pensabene Hearn**
EDITOR, ONLINE AND PRINT **Meredith Barrett**	EDITORIAL DESIGNERS **Brian Ross, Ellie Jeon**
ASSOCIATE EDITOR **Rachel Corradetti**	PROP/WARDROBE STYLIST **Kelsey-Lynn Corradetti**
ONLINE EDITOR **Kiersten Corradetti**	MARKETING COORDINATOR **Patricia D'Amato**
EDITORIAL ASSISTANTS **Sharlene Liladhar, Brittany Seki, Chelsea Kennedy**	SENIOR WEB DESIGNER **Chris Barnes**

IMPORTANT

The information in this book reflects the author's
experiences and opinions and is not intended to replace
medical advice.

Before beginning this or any nutritional or exercise
regimen, consult your physician to be sure it is
appropriate for you. Ask for a physical stress test.

Dedication

I dedicate this book to my daughter, Kiersten, who inspired me to break it down to just the rules!

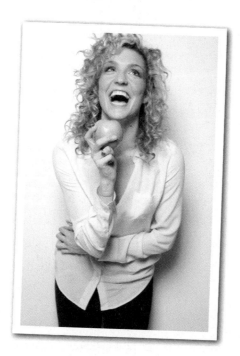

Contents

Make these changes · 58

Food basics · 84

Last words · 116

My
Aha!
moment

No More
Frustration!

It's time
to go
back to
basics!

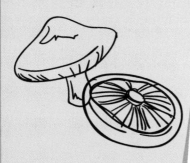

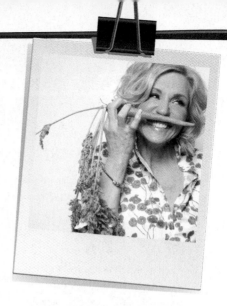

Introduction
Eat Real
Not Fake

Dear Dieter,

On a recent book promotional tour through far too many towns to remember, I had an Aha! moment. (I wonder if Oprah wishes she had copyrighted that term?) Anyway, I discovered something very important – I noticed members of the audience looking confused when I suggested various ways to change one's lifestyle. For example, I would mention ditching sugar, then adding flaxseed, then eating five or six meals each day, oh and don't forget water. As one seminar followed another, I realized I was overwhelming these lovely people. And as friendly as I have tried to make *The Eat-Clean Diet®* series, I also understand reading a 250+ page book on nutrition can be overwhelming, too.

That's when it hit me. I needed to write a simple, fun, upbeat and portable book that would serve as a guide to help people begin embracing the *Eat-Clean Diet* lifestyle. I realized I may not be getting my message across in the most accessible way. Forgive me; nutrition is my life's passion, and I tend to get too excited by the little details. It's time to go back to basics!

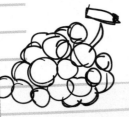

Just the Rules is that tool for you: the busy mom, truck driver, traveling sales executive, author, athlete, priest, student or whatever your job description may be. You're short on time and low on attention span though you want to do the best for your family and yourself.

Though small, *Just the Rules* is packed with readily digestible information to help you get on the path to wellness. We condensed the information so you can pick up the book and get started no matter who or where you are. We have taken the frustration out of the process! My goal is to keep you from glazing over and to gently but firmly push you over the line to getting back the best version of you.

Remember who that is? It is you running, swimming, making love, dancing, playing with your kids and looking like life has blanketed you with radiant health and energy. People will notice and ask, "What is different about you? What have you done?" And you can whip out your little tool *Just the Rules* and say, "I learned how to Eat Clean and I love it!"

Remember,
I am always listening,

Tosca Reno

Eat like
a baby,
baby
basics!

Eat more
not less

What did
grandma eat?
And what did her
grandma eat?

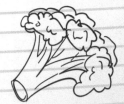

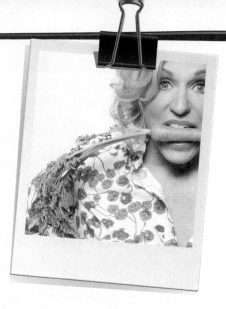

How to
Eat

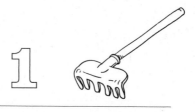

Our ancestors did it for us and before us

We have the cumulative knowledge and wisdom of many generations before us, so why do we choose to ignore it?

Our human race is a collection of our ancestors' DNA; we are part of all who have come before us. Our ancestors gained and left behind a great deal of knowledge regarding food. Just because they have passed doesn't mean we should turn up our noses at their legacy. Don't you want your children and their children to use the lessons you have taught them? Over the generations we have seen how ignoring such valuable information has affected our society; we have become polluted, material driven, inactive and unhealthy. And now we want a quick fix for it all!

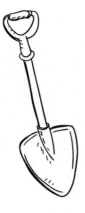

Our ancestors knew that all good things come with time, patience and hard work. This included cultivation of crops and food. A long time ago food was not as easy to come by as it is now. The Aztecs didn't just walk into a grocery store and pick out treats. Their food was planted, watered, dried by the sun, fertilized and prepared by hand. Food was meant and used to power the body, allowing it to function like a well-oiled machine. Industrialization and technology have removed these steps from our food production efforts. This is not all bad, of course. As much as we can thank our ancestors for hard organic work, we can also thank them for innovation, technology and industrialization. However, we must use modern innovation both wisely and in moderation.

I am not saying you personally should grow everything you eat because this isn't possible for most of us. The idea here is that our ancestors didn't sit on the couch plowing chips all day. They worked hard and rested and ate when and what they needed. They understood how to make food last rather than eating every last morsel in one sitting. We too need to adapt elements of this lifestyle into our own and use our resources appropriately!

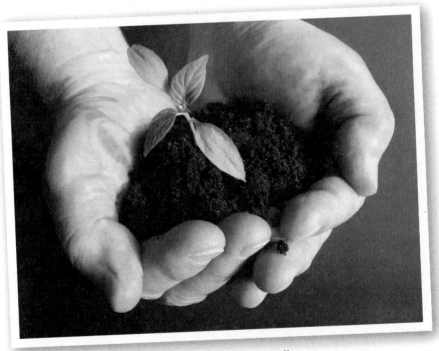

Our ancestors knew that all good things come with time, patience and hard work.

Eat more, not less

Contrary to common "diet" practices, including starving yourself and omitting entire food groups, Eating Clean allows you to eat more and weigh less by making informed food choices.

An *Eat-Clean Diet* follower knows to eat five or six small meals a day by choosing from a cornucopia of lean proteins (LP) and complex carbs (CC) (see Rule #40: LP + CC sitting in a tree, pg. 92) and by avoiding starchy, sugary, empty-calorie, industrialized and high-fat foods.

Eating several smaller meals of lean protein and complex carbs daily will fire up your metabolism, making you a highly functioning, fat-burning machine. Your entire body will thank you and you'll be amazed at how good you look and feel.

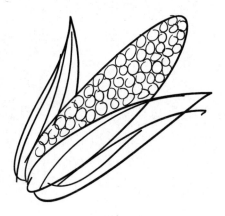

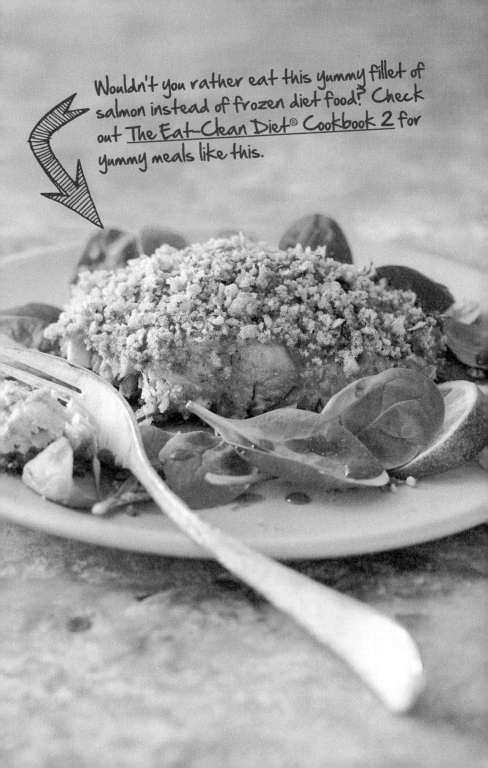

Wouldn't you rather eat this yummy fillet of salmon instead of frozen diet food? Check out _The Eat-Clean Diet® Cookbook 2_ for yummy meals like this.

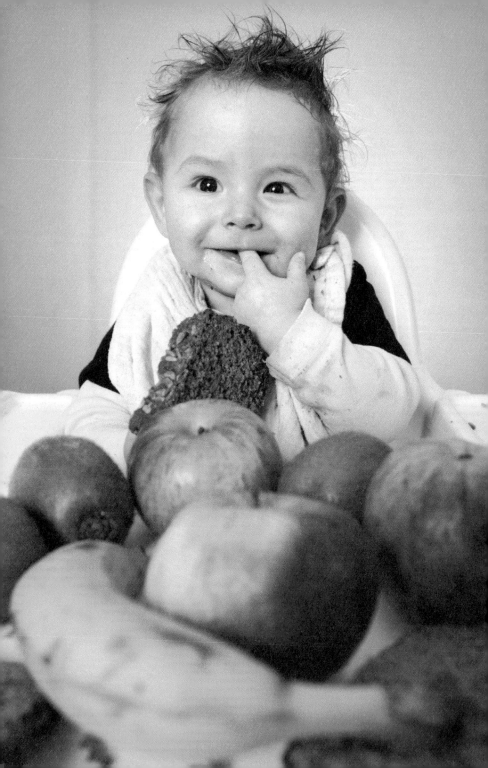

Eat like a baby, baby basics!

A baby's life is simple: sleep, cry, eat, sleep, cry, eat, sleep, cry, eat, sleep, cry, eat, and a lot of elimination – you get the point. Notice how many times a baby needs to eat? Pay attention – you should be eating this often too. Going back to the "basics" – the "baby basics" of eating and sleeping (and perhaps crying if you need to!) – is key to grasping the *Eat-Clean Diet* way of life.

When you Eat Clean, you know to eat every two to three hours to fuel a powerful, efficient, machine-like metabolism. If you don't feel hungry or you tend to forget to eat, schedule it on the clock: 7 am breakfast, 10 am snack, 1 pm lunch, 4 pm snack, 7 pm dinner and 10 pm snack if you need one. Hungry or not, stick to this plan; your body will reset and as a result kick-start your fat-burning abilities. Before long you won't need the reminder of the clock; your own body will tell you when it's time to eat. Remember to fuel your body with lean protein and complex carbs, not high-fat, starchy, sugary, empty-calorie foods.

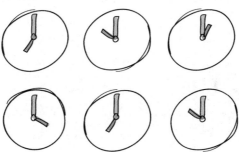

4

Break the fast

Are you connecting the dots? Break the fast = breakfast? It comes when you wake up from a seven- to eight-hour sleep, which means it's been a very long time since you've eaten, and then you break the fast by eating "breakfast." It should happen every morning, so why do some choose to skip it?

Eat-Clean Diet followers know you should always wake up to a sizeable breakfast because it is the first taste of food after a full night of rest and repair. Eating a healthy breakfast gets your whole system going – both your brain and body will work better, setting the tone for optimal performance and nutrition for the rest of the day.

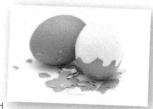

Having a full tummy first thing wards off all those sugar- and fat-laden junk food attacks. Why? Because you start your day off satisfied and full of nutritious and delicious food. Your body doesn't need to crave anything, because you've fed it well.

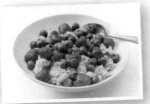

And the best breakfast award goes to … oatmeal. It's the champion of all breakfast foods because it regulates your blood sugar and keeps you fuller longer. One cup of oatmeal contains 8 grams of fiber – that's a full third of the dietary reference intake (DRI).

5

What did grandma eat? And what did her grandma eat?

I bet you can't really think back that far, but perhaps you could imagine. Picture your stereotypical white-haired and wrinkled grandma full of wise advice and all the answers. For the most part, this grandma has all the best information on nutrition.

Food was less processed and packaged and it was chemical free in the past. We should use these criteria for our own food choices. Our grandparents and great-grandparents had only real, whole, nutritious food. They had no processed or plastic alternatives. No gimmicks, no imposters – just the real deal. They also had tighter budgets, and a tighter budget meant less food, smaller portions and no overeating. This is the profile of Eating Clean – real, whole food and not too much of it.

Get in touch with your roots and eat them too!

6

Plan it!

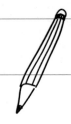

Tips to keep you on track

Turn to the clock to help keep your metabolism in check. Schedule your meals for exactly three hours apart. You will notice over time that your stomach will start reminding you every three hours that it is time to eat. You won't even need to look at the clock!

Another helpful tip is to keep a detailed food journal that includes portion sizes, when you have eaten and what you have eaten. *The Eat-Clean Diet®* *Companion* is the ideal place to start. Reflect on your journal entries every week and you will see if you are a true *Eat-Clean Diet* follower or not! You may be surprised to discover how many extras sneak their way into your meal plan, such as the second helping of risotto you just couldn't resist.

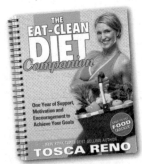

People who set plans like this are much more likely to stay on track and reach success.

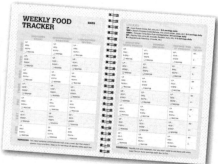

It's a goal!

Want the 50 percent advantage? Then write it down. Yes, folks who set goals and write them down are 50 percent more likely to succeed. Whip out a piece of paper right now and get started. A pencil might help too.

#1 What is your ultimate overall goal? This is important to help you visualize where you will be in the future.

#2 What goal would you like to achieve in the next week? Think of something like ditching cream in your coffee or cleaning out your fridge and restocking it with Eat-Clean foods.

#3 What goal would you like to achieve in the next month? Think of something like losing eight pounds.

#4 What goal would you like to achieve in six months? This could be a goal such as running your first 10 km race.

#5 What goal would you like to achieve in a year? This could be sticking to your ultimate goal or entering your first figure competition.

Set new weekly and monthly goals each week and month and stick to the changes you've made in the past. This way of goal setting will allow you to celebrate small victories, while also keeping you on track to achieve the bigger goal at hand.

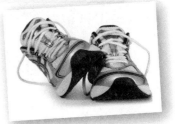

Color up!

Just like your wardrobe, your plate should never follow a tired, bland, monotonous color scheme. Incorporate bold colors into your meals. Choose foods that are naturally colored by the sun, soil and rain. The more color on your plate the healthier you will be! I often design my meal around colors. It's fun!

Real food is naturally colorful inside and out, while fake food is just bland with loud packaging. Opt for produce in a rainbow of colors: bright reds, oranges, yellows, greens, purples and varieties of brown.

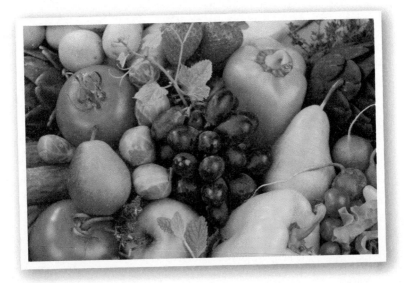

Eating colorful food offers numerous health benefits. These foods provide anti-aging properties, encourage weight loss and help ward off disease including cancer and diabetes. Each color group of food provides different benefits so be sure to include a spectrum of food hues in your eating. White and green produce offers immune-fighting properties. Red and blue fruits and vegetables promote healthy circulation, while yellow and orange foods strengthen your heart and purify your blood.

> Colorful foods are filled with more nutrients and flavor than bland, monotonous, processed foods. Let the food do the talking.

Drink the horta!

But wait? Doesn't horta mean greens? You want me to drink the greens?

In a way I do recommend you drink your greens, but not necessarily in a literal sense. Let me explain. Drinking the horta (for our purposes) means: drink the cooking water left over from boiling your vegetables. Need an example? If you boil or even steam broccoli, don't throw the cooking water down the sink; pour it in a glass and drink up! Or save it to make soup stock.

But why would you ever do that? You do this because when you boil vegetables, important vitamins and minerals are leached into the cooking water. Cooked vegetables are often (not always) left less nutritious than raw. Now the cooking water contains the good stuff. So don't turn up your nose when someone tells you to "drink the horta!"

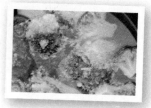

10

Eat more grass

At this point you probably think I'm nuts – drink the horta, eat a rainbow and now grass? Well a successful *Eat-Clean Diet* follower knows the stuff that comes from the ground is best for building a healthy, fit and fabulous body.

Grass is nutritious for everyone; the only problem is humans don't have the digestive equipment needed to break it down. We cannot just go outside and graze the fields. No cheeks full of green for us. Instead we have to get someone else to do that for us. Do you know what I am thinking of? Yes, it's a cow, a chicken, a bison, a deer … the list of grass eaters goes on and on. Try to ensure that the meat and dairy products you consume come from grass-fed animals.

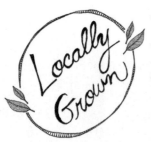

Why? Meat from grass-fed animals has less saturated fat and is lower in cholesterol and calories than meat from grain-fed animals. Grass-fed meat and dairy products also contain higher amounts of vitamins C and E, beta carotene and a number of health-promoting fats, including omega-3 fatty acids.

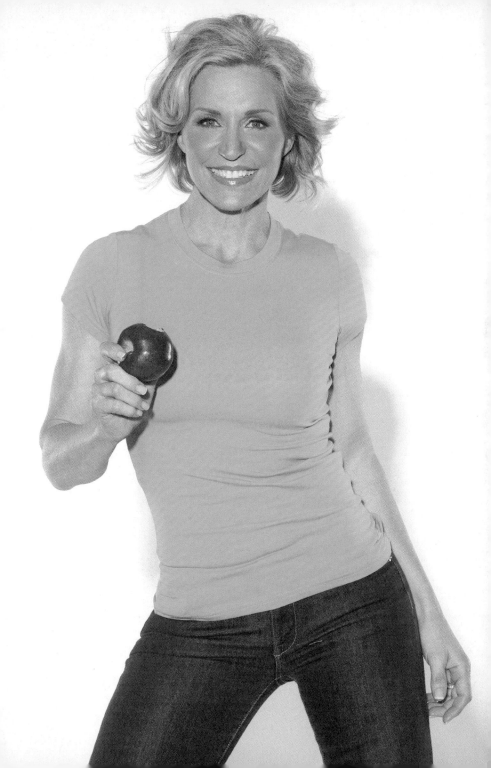

Let's not overlook the obvious here – these animals are meant to eat grass. It's in their biology to graze and digest the grassy fields that surround us – they even have a specialized enzyme and digestive system, for goodness' sake! When you select grass-fed meat and dairy products you are actually improving the welfare of the animal. Personally, you take action against the degradation of the environment. Economically, you promote local and small-scale businesses. Geographically, you aid the development of rural communities. And, best of all, you give yourself and your family the healthiest possible food. A win-win-win-win situation!

11

Eat living foods

Eating living foods means you are eating foods as close to their natural source as possible. Cracking open a can of Chef Boyardee or tearing the package off a Twinkie is the furthest thing from what I am imagining right now. Living foods have just been plucked from the ground, fished out of the water, laid in the nest or picked from the tree. These foods have the highest nutritional content and have been placed in your hand by the least amount of transportation. They are good for you and for the earth. For more details on how to attain the most from your living foods see Rules #27 (pg. 62), #28 (pg. 63), #29 (pg. 66) and #32 (pg. 71).

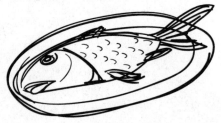

12

Smaller portions = smaller pants

Downsize your dinner plate!

You've been Eating Clean for weeks and months now but you're getting soooo frustrated that the weight isn't just falling off. "How come it is for everyone else? Why not me? I'm eating my five or six meals, I'm pairing LP and CC at every meal. I don't even cheat (or as I say, treat). I exercise three or four times a week and still the scale won't budge!"

It is possible to be an "over" Clean eater. You think, "Oh wow! I'm eating healthy foods; now I can eat even more!" Let's just stop right there: Yes you are making great food choices, and you are probably eating more than you used to, but that doesn't mean you can eat an infinite amount of it. Your body has a limit on its gas tank (stomach) and too much Clean fuel will build up and add fat. You need to get in tune with your body, your metabolism and your

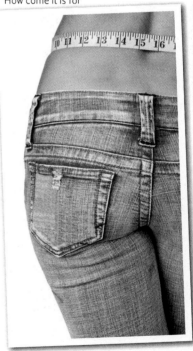

Are you hungry? Or are you thirsty?

stomach. Listen to your body's natural ability to tell you when you're full and when you're hungry. Even healthy foods need to be consumed in balance.

Perhaps, my friend, you need to take a look at your portion sizes. Learn to be mindful of how much food and ultimately how many calories you are putting into your stomach. Being mindful of how much you consume has nothing to do with calorie counting and everything to do with listening to your body – and really listening. I call this your "stomach sense." Are you hungry? Or are you thirsty? Listen to when you're full and listen to when you're hungry. Eat or don't eat according to the signals. In the beginning it is hard to determine what these signals are, and that is why one of your *Eat-Clean Diet*® Principles is to measure your food in the palm of your hand! Soon it will all become second nature.

1 serving lean protein =
palm of your hand

1 serving of complex carbs from
whole grains = one cupped hand

1 serving of complex carbs from
fresh fruits or vegetables =
two cupped hands together

Smaller portions allow your body to function on the fuel it actually needs and not the food you simply eat based on desire, meaning less is stored as fat. Lighten up your meals and you'll feel a lot lighter too – not to mention you will be in dire need of smaller pants!

Buddha called this "the middle way" and Goldilocks called it "just right." So just like Buddha and Goldilocks, do some metabolism meditation and find your Eat-Clean middle ground.

13

Fletcherize and swallow

Or you'll be a gobbling, gobbling glutton!

Does your food disappear off your plate faster than your Hoover picks up dust off your carpet? Do you wonder who the Houdini is behind your food disappearance? You might be a culprit of gobble, gobble glutton disorder. It's a very common disorder in today's fast-paced, fast-food nation.

This disorder classifies those eaters out there who don't take breaths or breaks between bites of food. Their food goes from lips to stomach without enough time to chew in between. Their fork races between their lips and plate at a rate similar to the ball in an Olympic table-tennis match. These people have few dinnertime conversations, always go back for seconds, are very vulnerable to choking and often finish meals feeling bloated and unsettled. Some of these people barely lift their heads from their plates. How did that meal end so quickly? Did they even taste it?

This non-medical disorder is easily treated. The treatment is called "fletcherizing." Chew, chew, chew, chew. Chew each food morsel 20 to 30 times before you swallow. Also, remind yourself to slooooowww down. There is no race when it comes to meals. Take a break, have a chat, have a sip of water and enjoy and savor the meal and the company.

Fletcherizing and slowing down will allow you to understand how full or empty your stomach is and will give your stomach the opportunity to properly digest your food. Ultimately you will downsize your dinner plate and maybe tighten that notch on your belt. Hello, smaller pants!

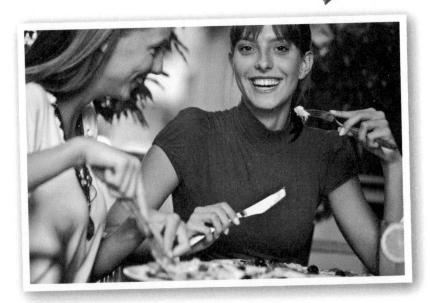

14

A treat is not a cheat ... a treat is a treat!

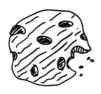

The Eat-Clean Diet® is a lifestyle choice, which means you adapt it to fit your life. If you must have birthday cake, then have it. Eating Clean is flexible, meaning you can celebrate – in moderation, and with thought.

Over time as an *Eat-Clean Diet* follower, you will easily apply an Eat-Clean lens to each meal of the day, allowing you to make intelligent decisions about eating. You will be able to look at a meal and decide whether or not it is "clean." The decision often comes down to: Clean foods you feel good about and not-so-Clean foods you know are not the best but still like to eat on occasion. The latter often get a bad rap and are referred to as "cheats."

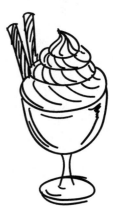

Cheats are feared by dieters! When you "cheat" you become overwhelmed with guilt and heartbreak. You've let yourself down and feel like a failure. These circumstances can even take over your psyche, leading you into a downward spiral where your cheats happen each day or even each meal, ruining any progress you have made and causing you to throw in the towel. But this doesn't have to happen.

First of all, let's change our thinking. We're going to call unclean foods "treats" instead of "cheats."

Why? Because "treat" is a much nicer word that doesn't hold any negative connotations. Treats are simply unclean foods you may choose to eat on occasion, but they won't hinder your success in the long run because you will pick up right where you left off once you've eaten them. For this reason treats are okay, but only every once in a while. What we need to be conscious of is how often we choose to enjoy a treat.

Treats present themselves all the time – in fact, sometimes they seem to appear around every corner – but you do have the willpower to turn them down if you plan for it. Allow yourself one treat each week. Choose which treat you will have. Enjoy it! But you don't have to make a whole meal of it. Perhaps you enjoy a glass of red wine with your meal on a Friday night. But because you've had a glass doesn't mean it's okay to have glass after glass. Or maybe you look forward to a dessert after a week of Eating Clean. Have the dessert, but don't decide to then eat a carton of ice cream!

With this attitude, the unclean food is no longer feared and can be enjoyed. You know that this treat does not in any way affect your regular meal choice. Moreover, this one delicious treat has not sabotaged your progress. In fact, it may fuel your Eat-Clean fire!

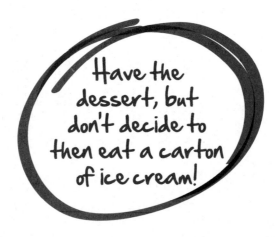

Have the dessert, but don't decide to then eat a carton of ice cream!

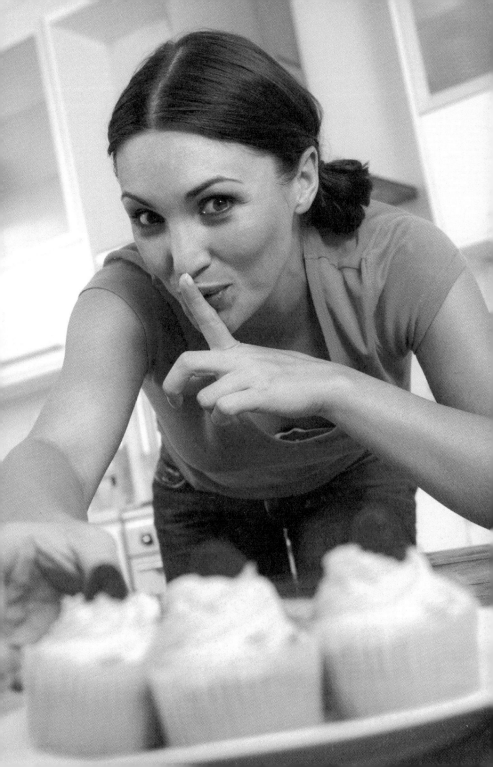

15

Your Aha! moment

Give yourself permission to change

This is the moment you realize you are on your way. For me this moment came after seeing a picture of my blobby self with my healthy, fit kids. I realized I wasn't going to be around to see them grow up if I didn't get my act together. For you, it could happen while you're trying on last year's bikini wondering why it doesn't fit, or when you're at the doctor's office receiving a piece of bad news about your health. Either way, it will happen. And that will be the moment when you give yourself permission to change. Don't ignore this moment. Grab it full on by the horns and run with it until you have achieved your goals. Your Aha! is the door opening into the life of the person you were always meant to be. Your Aha! is the first step into the future.

Before,
age 39

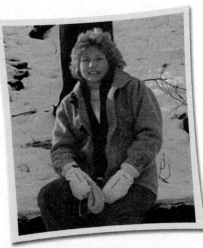

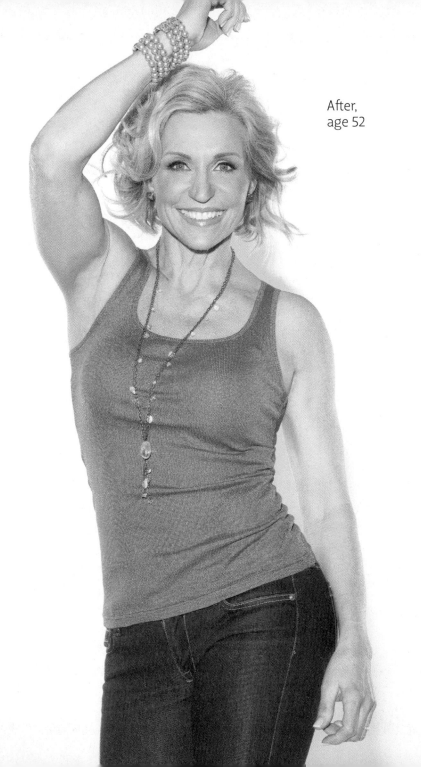

After,
age 52

Can't read it? Don't eat it!

Diet Foods Make You FAT!

Good Carbs, Bad Carbs

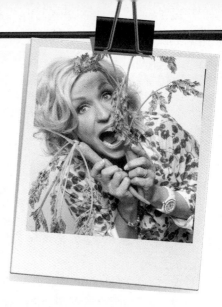

False
Advertising

16

Can't read it?
Don't eat it!

There are two crucial food-labeling rules to follow:

 # 1 Read labels.

 # 2 If the label contains words that look like they're from chemistry class, leave it on the shelf!

Why would you put something in your body that you can't pronounce, let alone fathom where it might have come from?

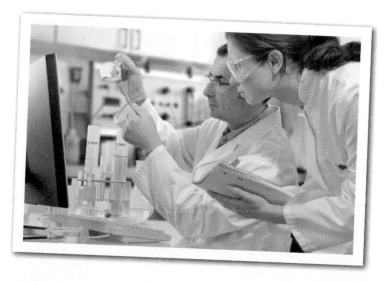

Although it might seem obvious, chemicals aren't food for you or any other living thing. Food scientists are paid big money to create long-lasting, artificially delicious food. Chemical concoctions become the prime ingredients in food on grocery store shelves, meaning a mad scientist is your own personal chef. It is no big surprise that money is enough motivation for food companies to ignore the negative impacts these chemicals have on your long-term health. Thus marketing people and food scientists come together to sell you some cleverly chemically concocted corporate dish. Yum!

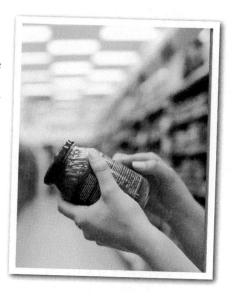

Massive food businesses are leading you blindly into a world of plastic food that will ultimately destroy your health, leaving you poor and them laughing all the way to the bank.

Chemicals aren't nutrition. They don't satisfy your hunger, they're addictive and they'll leave you sick in the hospital with one of the many all too prevalent North American chronic diseases including diabetes or cancer.

So I'll repeat:

 # 1 Read labels.

#2 If the label contains words that look like they're from chemistry class, leave it on the shelf!

17

New and improved!

You're not moved.

Have you ever watched *Mad Men*? Well if you haven't, I advise you to watch at least one episode to understand that we are all guilty of falling for a cleverly campaigned product through advertising. One word:

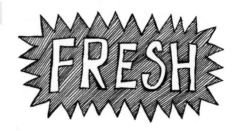

"new," "fresh," "organic" or "green" can immediately alter our impression of the product even if the product wasn't actually changed. I guarantee you that whatever the word, it's just marketing to a trend and in most cases the product hasn't changed.

Don't be fooled by advertising and marketing tricks. Words such as "diet," "organic" and "added nutrients" are simply tools to entice the consumer to purchase these products. It's a gimmick and *Eat-Clean Diet* followers are no longer naïve – we know how to research our food in our quest to find real nutrition, leaving pretty plastic packaging and unrecognizable ingredients behind.

An *Eat-Clean Diet* follower wants the real food deal: easy-to-read labels, see-through packaging or no packaging at all and five or fewer ingredients ... preferably only one ingredient. It truly is best to eat the foods you can easily identify. These are honest foods – no tricks or gimmicks!

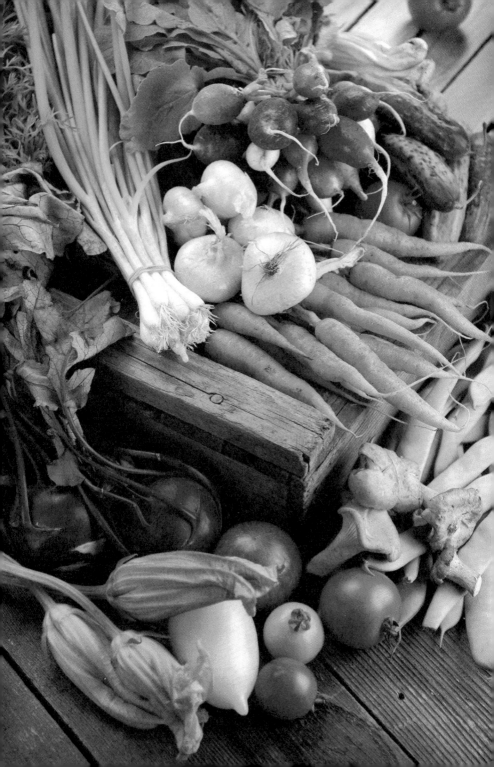

18

Beware of everlasting foods

A short lifespan for them means a long lifespan for you!

With few exceptions (oats, brown rice, oils), products with a long shelf life do not provide nutrition. The longer the shelf life, the less these products even resemble nutrition. They are just your next ticket to a hospital room.

Most perishable foods come with an expiry date. Think of bread, milk, meats, cheese, etc. These foods will go bad in a relatively short time. Oftentimes, processed foods such as Twinkies and crackers have expiry dates so far into

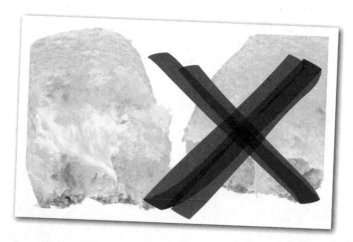

Nutritional Information
for Snack Cakes

Nutrition Facts

Serving Size 1 cake (42.5 g)

Amount Per Serving

Calories 150	Calories from Fat 41
	% Daily Value*
Total Fat 4.5g	**7%**
Saturated Fat 2.5g	**13%**
Trans Fat 0.0g	
Cholesterol 20mg	**7%**
Sodium 220mg	**9%**
Total Carbohydrates 27.0g	**9%**
Sugars 18.0g	
Protein 1.0g	

Vitamin A 0%	•	Vitamin C 0%
Calcium 0%	•	Iron 2%

* Based on a 2000 calorie diet

INGREDIENTS: ENRICHED BLEACHED WHEAT FLOUR [FLOUR, FERROUS SUL-
FATE, "B" VITAMINS (NIACIN, THIAMINE MONONITRATE (B1), RIBOFLAVIN (B2),
FOLIC ACID)], SUGAR, CORN SYRUP, WATER, HIGH FRUCTOSE CORN SYRUP,
PARTIALLY HYDROGENATED VEGETABLE SHORTENING (CONTAINS ONE OR
MORE OF: SOYBEAN, CANOLA OR PALM OIL), DEXTROSE, WHOLE EGGS. CON-
TAINS 2% OR LESS OF: MODIFIED CORNSTARCH, CELLULOSE GUM, WHEY,
LEAVENINGS (SODIUM ACID PYROPHOSPHATE, BAKING SODA, MONOCALCIUM
PHOSPHATE), SALT, CORNSTARCH, CORN FLOUR, CORN DEXTRINS, MONO AND
DIGLYCERIDES, POLYSORBATE 60, SOY LECITHIN, NATURAL AND ARTIFICIAL
FLAVORS, SOY PROTEIN ISOLATE, SODIUM STEAROYL LACTYLATE, SODIUM
AND CALCIUM CASEINATE, CALCIUM SULFATE, SORBIC ACID (TO RETAIN
FRESHNESS), COLOR ADDED (YELLOW 5, RED 40). MAY CONTAIN PEANUTS
OR TRACES OF PEANUTS.

the future that one box might sit on the shelf for months. How? Because they are packed with preservatives to keep them around for a long, long time. A distant expiry date means this product isn't going bad for a long time and, guess what folks, real food goes bad!

Keep in mind that foods found in the produce section, such as greens, vegetables and fruit – anything fresh – will not have a clearly labeled expiration date. But leave these foods out on your counter for only a short time and they will go bad. Bacteria attack the organic particles of the food, giving off a pungent aroma we've probably all smelled coming from our fridge or countertop at one time or another. Bacteria are smart enough to recognize real food, and we should be too!

So buy products with a short lifespan and see yours increase by years!

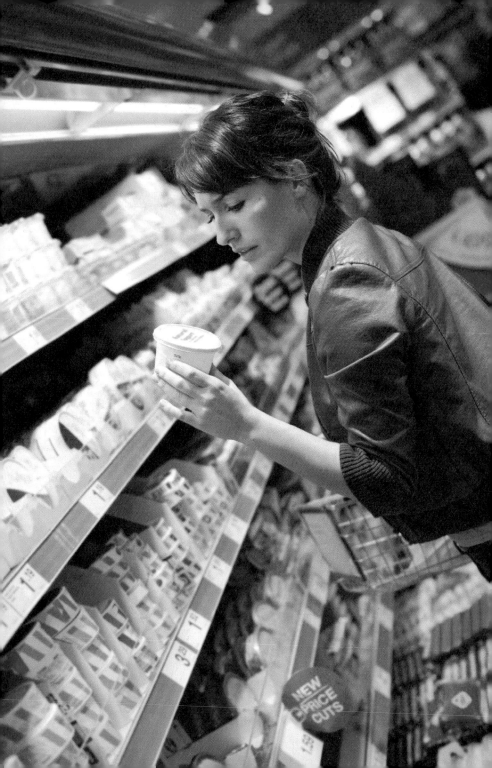

19

"Food" is not food: a discussion on anti-food

Just because you are in a grocery store surrounded by "food" does not mean you can assume what you see is actually real food. Bright packages, nutrition labels, marketing claims, gizmos, plastic prizes, lists of ingredients and more will confuse you into thinking you are purchasing food. But beware! Much of what is in your local grocery store is not real food!

Much like Rule #16, if you can't decipher the ingredients on what you are about to buy then leave it. Some food items are more like science experiments than natural, earth-grown nutrition. Best to stick to what you can see and what you can read. "Foods" that are more like science experiments are what I refer to as "anti-foods." Anti-foods normally have more than five ingredients, and many of those ingredients are either unpronounceable chemicals, hydrogenated fats or some sort of sugar.

Anti-foods are "displacing foods of modern commerce," according to Lierre Keith, author of *The Vegetarian*

Take a stand for your health and your wallet, even for the earth.

Myth. Industrialized foods take the place of nutrient-dense, whole foods, robbing us of the nutrients required for optimal health.

Don't give in! Take a stand for your health and your wallet, even for the earth. Support those who want to give you real food – they won't lie to you; they'll simply sell you a genuine, wholesome and delicious product.

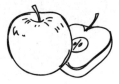

Diet foods make you fat

Clean foods keep you lean!

Have you noticed that when you attempt to go on a "diet" you end up losing a few pounds only to gain them all back plus five pounds more? Diet foods don't make you leaner; they make you fatter than you already are!

Want to know why? It's all in the word "diet." The word itself is a clever marketing tool causing people to buy the stuff and making them crazy because they confuse healthy eating with dieting. Diet products are often

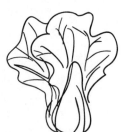

obese with chemicals, additives and sugar, leaving you void of nutrition. The word "diet" gives you false hope and the permission to give in to cravings and indulgences because at the end of the day you can always say, "Well, I ate diet chips and diet cookies!" Diet foods don't make you accountable – they make you fat.

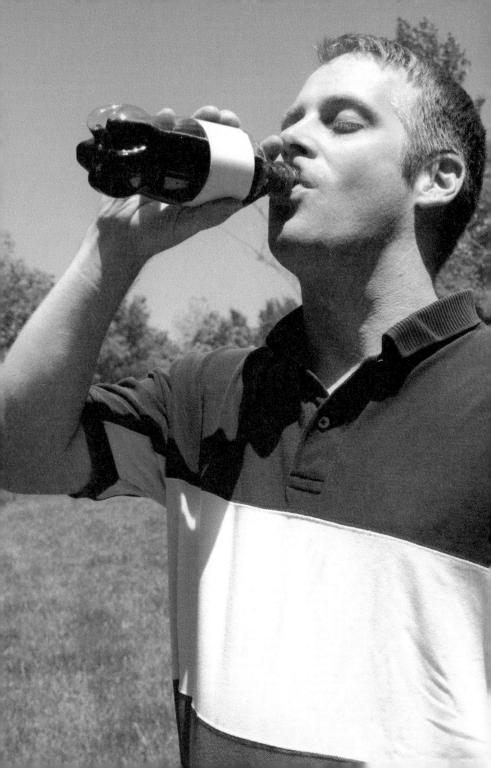

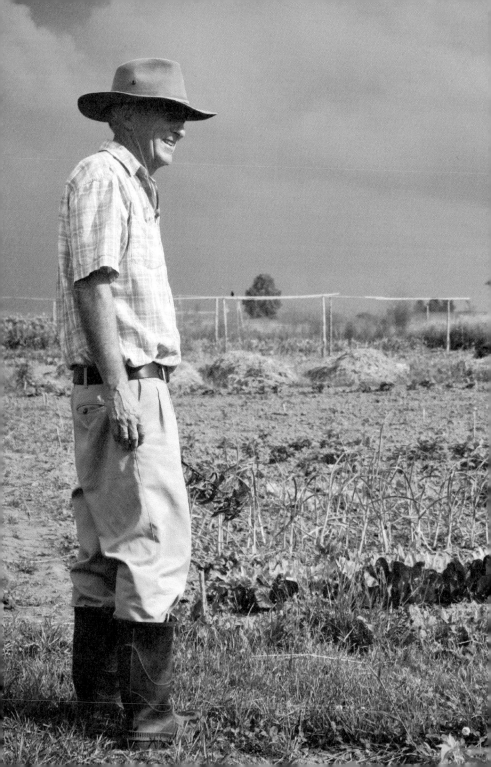

21

Beware the suits!

Seek out the flannels!

In this book of rules we have discussed quite a few times that heavily pack-aged, loud, advertised foods are often fake foods. These fake foods make you sick, fat and unhealthy. These foods, however, are far more accessible than most healthy foods. How does this happen, you ask? How could the most accessible foods be the ones that make you sick? Who is responsible for this? Well, I like to call them "the suits" – the scientists, marketers, clever businessmen and investors. The suits don't care about their consumer, but they do care a great deal about money. They bring in loads of revenue at your expense. Do your research on the foods and companies you may buy food from and discover who the suits are. Learn which marketing tools they're using on you and learn how to make to the healthiest decisions for you. The products the suits create generally loiter around the center aisles of your grocery store and always have five or more ingredients including those you cannot pronounce – oh, and sugar, too.

Seek out "the flannels" instead. And by that I mean those humble hard-working, flannel-shirt-wearing farmers who bring you fresh produce at a low cost. I recommend sticking to the outside perimeter of the grocery store, where the flannels have their products. Always do your research, shop local before organic and try to get information straight from the source. If you have the opportunity, shop at farmers' markets. Ask them questions about their produce, growing and harvesting procedures and what they feed their cattle, pigs and poultry. Be inquisitive and always beware the suits!

22

Is bread a food group?

Is Cheez Whiz cheese? The answer is no! But it seems one of the hardest things for people to let go of is their bread, bread, bread! Let me tell you now, people, bread does little more for your body than give it a giant dose of sugar and often a big tummy ache. If we think back to days long past, bread was a somewhat Eat-Clean food. It was made with four simple ingredients – water, whole wheat flour, yeast and a little salt. Now we have turned bread into some sort of science experiment. From zillions of preservatives to a giant dose of bleaching, most bread offers little more than a spoonful of sugar. That is, unless you go back to your roots (as outlined in Rule #5, pg. 21). Make your own bread. It's not hard to do and the aroma seeping from your oven will definitely attract attention. You can also purchase sprouted grain breads, like my favorite, Ezekiel. It's made just as it was years ago. Now this bread is a food! Everything about it is Clean and it will fill you with nutrition. As with any grain product, though, bread must be consumed in moderation. And for ultimate weight control, keep it out of your diet altogether – especially the white stuff!

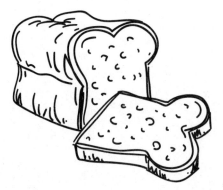

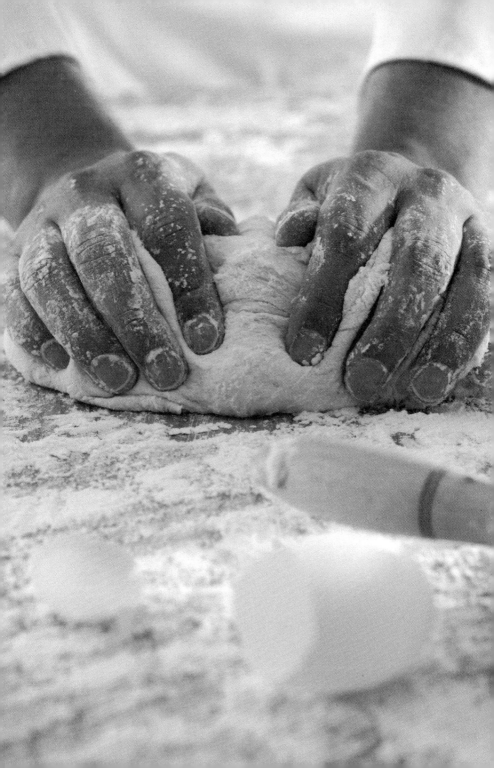

23

Good carbs, bad carbs

Carbohydrates have gotten a bad rap! Too bad because, along with protein and fat, carbs are a macronutrient essential to the body. Your brain loves carbs. Just try going without and see if you can operate your cell phone. So what's the problem?

We are gorging on processed carbohydrates. Our grocery-store shelves are full of them and our snack bars and coffee shops offer little more. Made from processed grains that lend very little nutritional value to our meals and send our blood sugar through the roof, these are the bad guys. Any excess carbohydrates are also stored as fat.

Good carbohydrates, on the other hand, are full of extra nutritional gems like fiber, vitamins and minerals, meaning they do a lot more for your body than a bowl full of white pasta ever will. They balance out your blood sugar and help your body use energy efficiently. So what are the good carbs? Vegetables, fruit, legumes and whole grains like brown rice and quinoa. And what are the bad carbs? Anything containing refined white flours and sugars. Stay away!

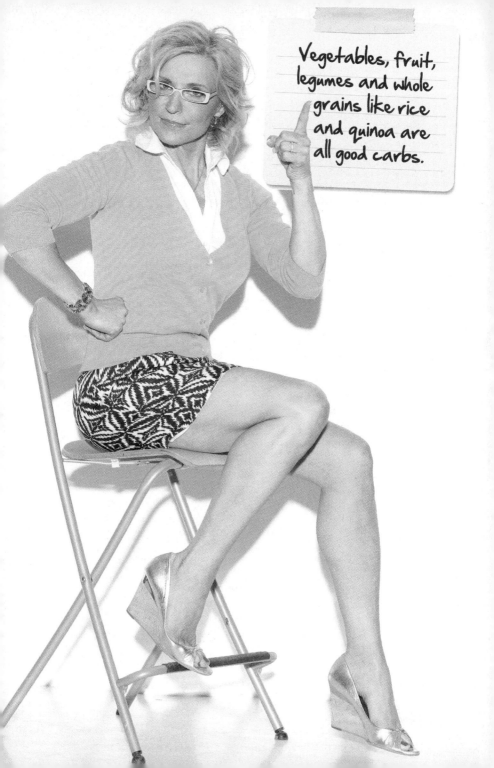

24

Where sugar is hiding

Everything you eat turns into glucose in your body so you can use it for every activity you do. The danger is, sugar is a refined anti-food. A scientist somewhere thought up the "brilliant" idea of sucking out the glucose and fructose from naturally sweet fruits and vegetables and using it to sweeten other things like soda, cookies and cakes. Think of an orange. This is a fruit naturally full of fructose. When you eat a piece of orange you give your body fiber, vitamin C and a host of other goodies found only in the whole orange. All of these things help your body use every ounce of nourishment from the orange before storing it as fat. The same is not true of a glass of orange juice. Instead you get all the sugar, very little fiber and fewer vitamins. Now your body reacts quickly to the sugars and stores them as fat. So sugar in its full-fruit form is great – in its processed, white, syrupy or juice form, not so great!

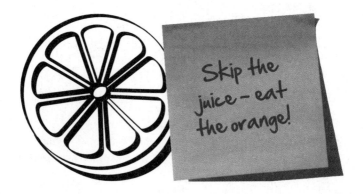

Skip the juice – eat the orange!

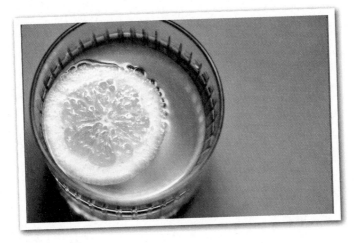

25

When is a detox not a detox?

This question seems ridiculous, as if I may have lost my marbles, but you heard it here first: Undergoing a detox can be downright dangerous if your pathways of elimination are not open. What pathways? Your bowels need to be moving, your kidneys need to be clean and able to flush urine, your lungs and nose need to be clear and you need to be able to sweat. Otherwise those toxins you are relocating from inside of you will simply be dumped elsewhere in your body and will make matters worse. Be smart; check your pathways and then detox. Support the process by drinking plenty of water energized with a pinch of sea salt and a squirt of fresh lemon juice.

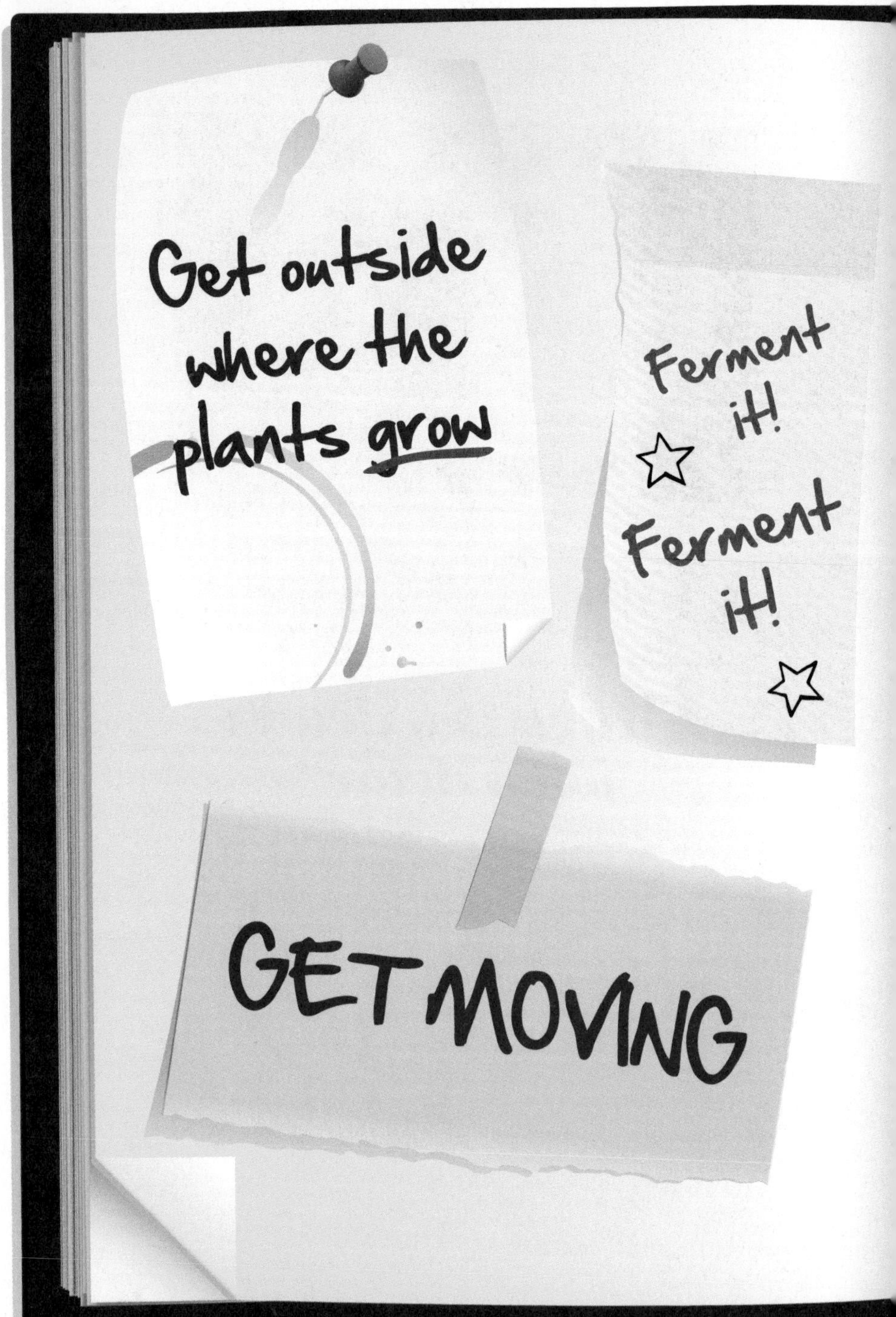

Get outside
where the
plants grow

Ferment
it!
☆
Ferment
it!
☆

GET MOVING

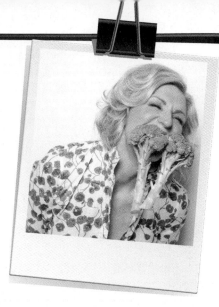

Make These Changes

Shopping challenge

Can you do your grocery shopping by purchasing food products with just five ingredients or fewer? I'm putting you up to the challenge! Try it, at least once, and I bet you'll never look back. Refer to Rule #16 (pg. 40) for the reasons why!

The rules of the challenge: purchase foods from your grocery store with only five ingredients or fewer.

Here's an Eat-Clean Diet tip:

★ **APPLE** = 1 ingredient ... apple

★ **OATMEAL** = 1 ingredient ... oats (*and I do not mean that individually packaged/flavored/instant oatmeal; I mean whole oats.*)

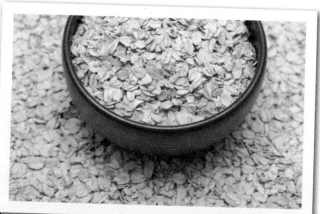

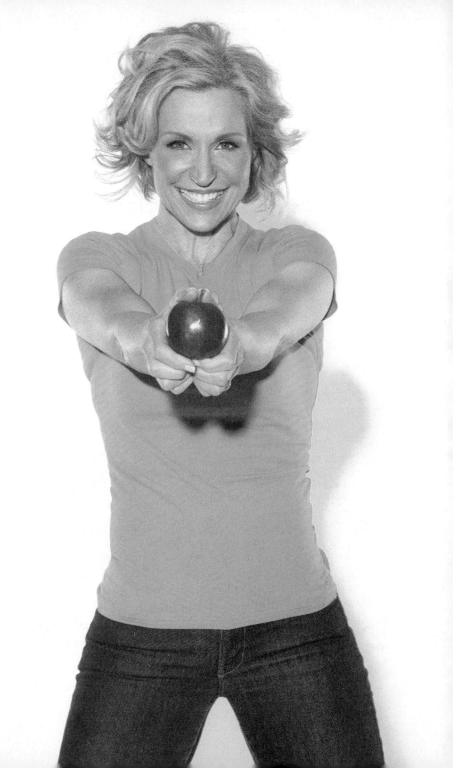

27

Get outside where the plants grow

Harmonize with your food. This means your food should come from a place where you can see it grow. Seeing, in an Eat-Clean world, is believing. To see where the food action happens will leave you enlightened about what you are putting in your mouth. It will teach you how it grows, swims, walks or flies, and what goes into the process: dirt, sun, rain, everything. Get this good stuff in you. It's hard to harmonize with a concrete factory, plastic products and

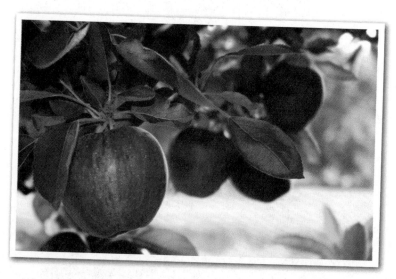

barrels of chemicals. Not to mention, you probably won't be allowed inside to harmonize with your food – you certainly won't be getting in touch with your man-made side. You are made in nature and nature provides what you need.

So try it! Get outside, plant a garden or go to a farm or a farmers' market. Visit a fish farm or a bison ranch (notice they eat grass). Grow or get close to the food you plan to eat so you can connect with the people you know have put effort into growing your food with their own hands, from the elements of the earth.

This is the stuff that will fill you with nutrition straight from the earth to your mouth.

This is the stuff an *Eat-Clean Diet* follower wants.

28

Can it, freeze it, dry it

... Harvest it, save it, pickle it!

Tired of seeing your fresh produce go bad and tossing your hard-earned pennies into the trash? Start saving your produce and your money by preserving your fresh food.

Preservation of food through the processes of pickling, drying, canning, freezing and, most recently, vacuum packing and dehydration will stop spoilage, allowing your once-fresh produce to always be fresh, last you all season and save you money, too.

It may seem like you're running backwards into ancient history, but this simple process will allow you to Eat Clean all year long without any excuses (It's too snowy, I have no money, I hate the grocery store … blah blah blah).

Become savvy in the preservation of your produce and you'll be making inexpensive yet exquisite Eat-Clean meals even into those bitter winter months.

Tips for successful freezing:

★ Produce freezes best if you cut it up beforehand

★ Bag or seal the chopped produce in an airtight container

★ To avoid frostbite on fresh produce, try to remove as much air from the container or plastic bag as possible

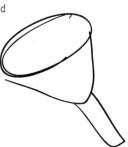

Canning and pickling 101:

★ Pickling means to immerse food into acidic or sugary liquid. The acids or sugars prevent bacteria from getting at the food, thus preserving it.

★ Canning means to give an airtight seal and a quick scalding. This prevents airborne bacteria from getting in the container in the first place.

★ Fermentation produces alcohol and other long-keeping foods like kimchi, which are staples in many healthy homes. For more about fermentation, see Rule #29 (pg. 66).

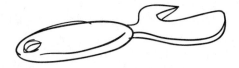

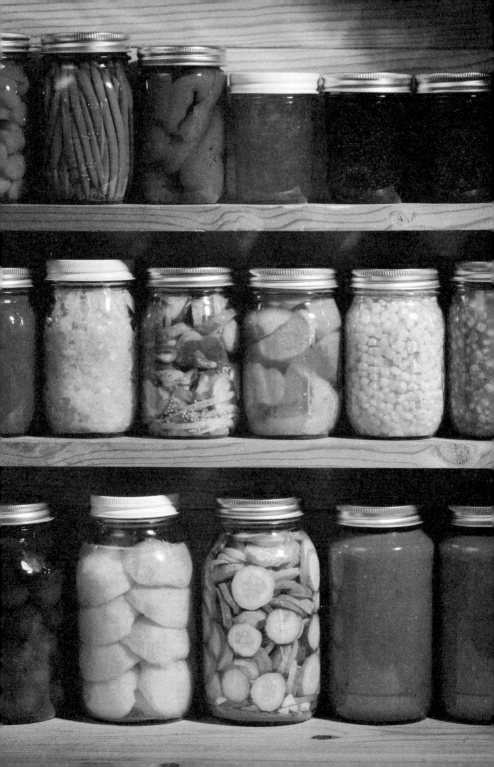

29

Ferment it

Another way to get the most out of food is to ferment it. Early cultures made and consumed fermented foods regularly. You can't blame them, can you? A fridge is hard to cart around and didn't even exist back then! The process of introducing friendly bacteria into foods, including milk, cheese, sauerkraut, beer and so on, not only makes them taste fabulous but also preserves them. Kind of handy when you need to stock up for the winter and have no other way to keep your food. But there is more! The friendly bacteria, primarily lactobacilli, help to predigest food, making it easier to digest and releasing more nutrients. It's a win-win – healthy food that tastes fantastic.

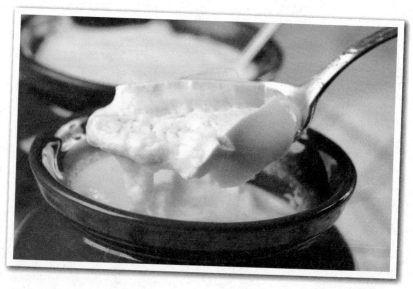

30

No plant boosters?

Just use poop!

And get your head out of the toilet! By plant boosters I mean fertilizer and by poop I mean manure. Instead of using fertilizer on your vegetable garden, use manure and save yourself from being infused with chemicals from your homegrown goods.

Bottom line: Most fertilizers are listed as toxic, so imagine what they will do to you. Among other things, they will store in your fat cells and accumulate as you consume more and more. Slowly you will become toxic yourself, which could lead to any number of diseases!

Quick facts on natural fertilizers:

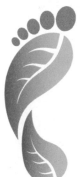

★ Organic fertilizers include animal manures, compost, bone meal and blood meal.

★ The natural environment can break these down and absorb them more readily than it can with artificial fertilizers.

★ Organic fertilizers like these contain microorganisms, helping plants assimilate the nutrients while also strengthening the plant's resistance to disease and pests.

★ Organic plant material helps to break down old plant material and return nutrients to the soil.

Caution: Organic fertilizers may leach into your water supply if used incorrectly.

31

'Tis the season to eat in season

Eat and buy local!

Eat local and in season all year 'round and you will drastically decrease the amount of money you spend while dramatically increasing the amount of nutrition you obtain from foods! Local, in-season foods are a) cheaper (and you support local business at the same time), and b) more nutritious because they spend less time in transit and more time being popped right into your mouth at their most vital peak. Recall Rule #11 (pg. 28).

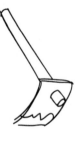

Eating local and in season is easy during the spring, summer and fall when farmers' fields are bursting with goodness. Visit local markets or farms in your area. However, you might be thinking: "How is eating this way possible when there is snow and ice on the ground?" Indeed, eating seasonally throughout the winter is more challenging, but there are plenty of foods that store well through the winter months. All you have to do is plan. Stockpile fresh produce from harvesting months in the summer and up into the fall.

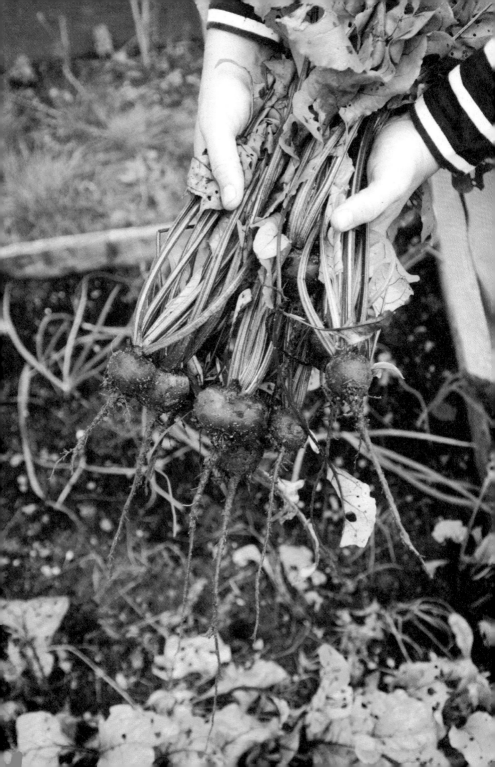

Recall Rule #28 (pg. 63), where we taught you the benefits of preserving. Apply this rule and you will never have to worry about spending loads of money on imported fruits and vegetables. You can also rest easy knowing that the foods coming from your neighborhood are far more nutritious than the produce coming from South America on gas-guzzling ships, trains, planes or automobiles with a huge carbon footprint.

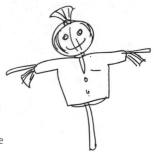

Test it out! Over the spring, summer and fall start shopping at local farmers' markets, at farms or in your own garden. Purchase (or grow) double the amount you usually would. Invest in a large deep freezer and start freezing or preserving (canning or pickling) half of your produce. It may take a couple of seasons to get your food quantities figured out, but once you do, you will find it was well worth the work. Some families enjoy using a food dehydrator, too. Figure out what works for you, use it and benefit from it.

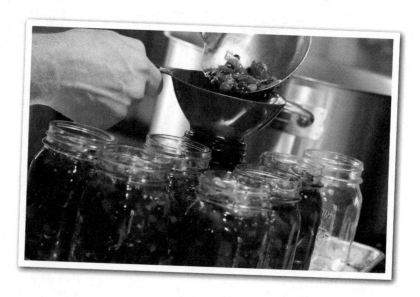

Let's analyze the wins to eating in-season:

★ You'll lower your food bills

★ You'll reduce your carbon footprint

★ You'll be supporting local business

★ You'll be the most healthy, Eat-Clean machine

★ You'll strengthen your immune system

Grow it, pick it, clean it, eat it!

Food should be grown, picked, chewed and swallowed.

If you have the space, opt for a vegetable garden. Not only will it save you money, it will decrease your carbon footprint, give you wonderfully nutritious food and get you out of the house and back to nature. Growing a vegetable garden can be relaxing and rewarding and gets you back in synch with what real food is.

Start off small with herbs, a tomato plant, a cucumber plant and a bean stalk. Then expand to carrots, lettuce, rhubarb, blueberries or whatever produce you want to eat! All you need is earth, manure for fertilizer, water, sun, dirt and a little elbow grease.

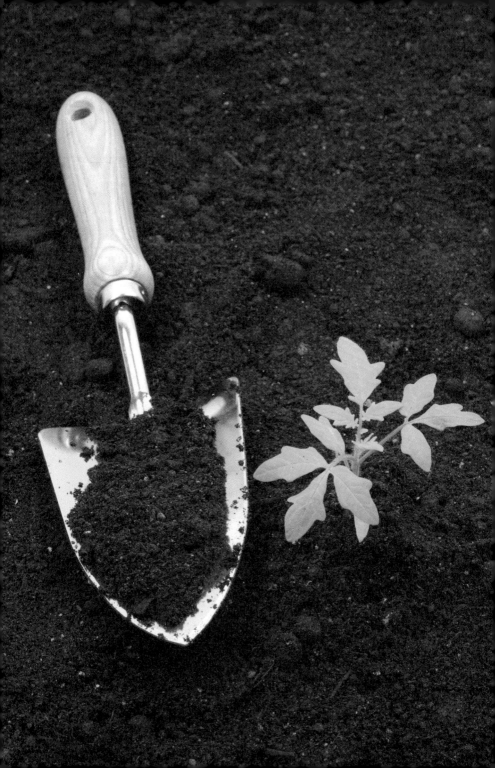

Even if you live in an apartment, you can grow vegetables on your balcony. Don't have a balcony? Many cities have communal garden options where you can rent a small plot.

Just remember this simple chant:

Grow it, pick it, clean it, eat it. Grow it, pick it, clean it, eat it. Grow it, pick it, clean it, eat it. Grow it, pick it, clean it, eat it.

For more information see Rules #27: Get outside where the plants grow (pg. 62), #28: Can it, freeze it, dry it (pg. 63), #30: No plant boosters? (pg. 67) and #31: 'Tis the season to eat in season (pg. 68).

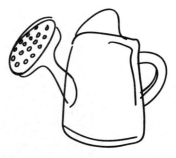

33

Learn how to cook

For some this may seem like a no-brainer, but many people find cooking a daunting task. Other people don't want to take the time, and some don't want to shop for the ingredients. Some people who don't cook just suffer from a lack of motivation, especially if they have no one for whom to do the cooking. My daughter hates to cook for herself. Her reasoning is: "It's just me, and I don't care." She'd settle for half an avocado and a slice of toast for any meal. I encourage you, for the benefit of your health, to please learn how to cook!

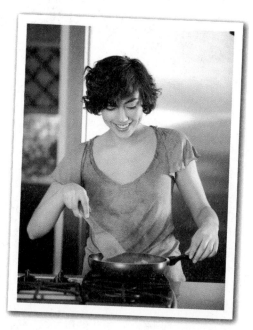

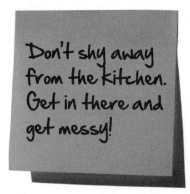

Don't shy away from the kitchen. Get in there and get messy!

Cooking is easy once you learn to relax and not worry about how good or bad your dish is going to turn out. Take a cooking class, watch The Food Network and buy lots of recipe books that interest you. Try out your skills and cook a new recipe every week. Experiment with Clean ingredients and embrace the limitless opportunity there is with food. You would be amazed at how little you have to fuss with Mother Nature's real food.

When you do the cooking you completely control what you are putting into your recipes. You can use the cleanest ingredients and know that you are making the best food for your optimal health. Cooking can be relaxing and enjoyable once you get the hang of it.

Once you've mastered your cooking prowess, pass on your skills! Teach your friends and family (especially your children if you have them) 10 Clean meals. This will encourage them to embrace Eating Clean and help them have the same optimal health you are working toward.

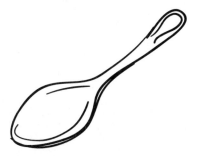

34

On the go? Take these!

Life is crazy for this on-the-move society. Don't want to undo your Eat-Clean handiwork? Reach for these top favorite quickie meals every time:

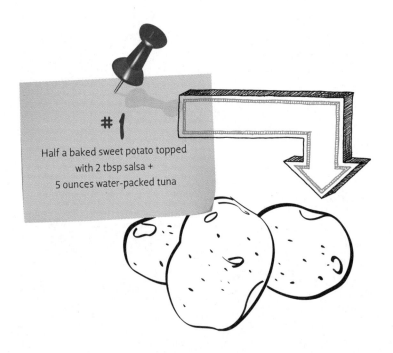

#1

Half a baked sweet potato topped
with 2 tbsp salsa +
5 ounces water-packed tuna

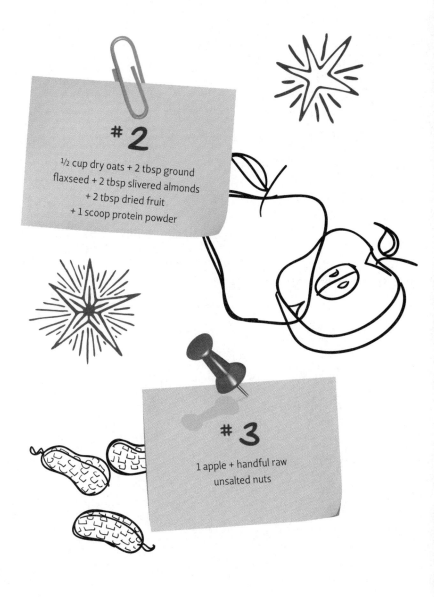

2

½ cup dry oats + 2 tbsp ground
flaxseed + 2 tbsp slivered almonds
+ 2 tbsp dried fruit
+ 1 scoop protein powder

3

1 apple + handful raw
unsalted nuts

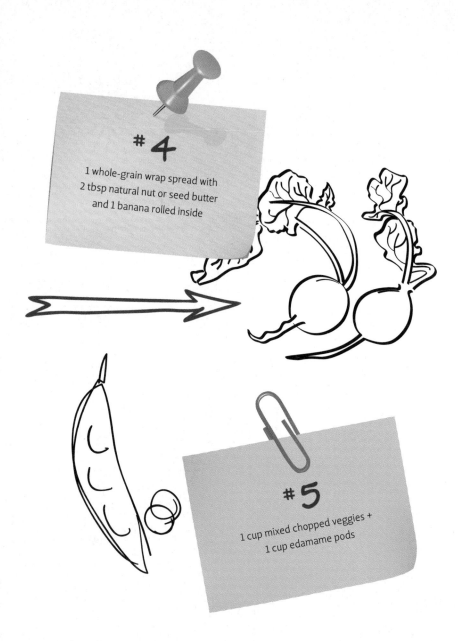

4

1 whole-grain wrap spread with
2 tbsp natural nut or seed butter
and 1 banana rolled inside

5

1 cup mixed chopped veggies +
1 cup edamame pods

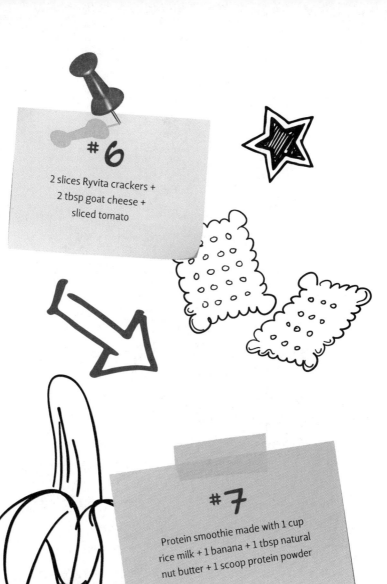

6

2 slices Ryvita crackers +
2 tbsp goat cheese +
sliced tomato

7

Protein smoothie made with 1 cup
rice milk + 1 banana + 1 tbsp natural
nut butter + 1 scoop protein powder

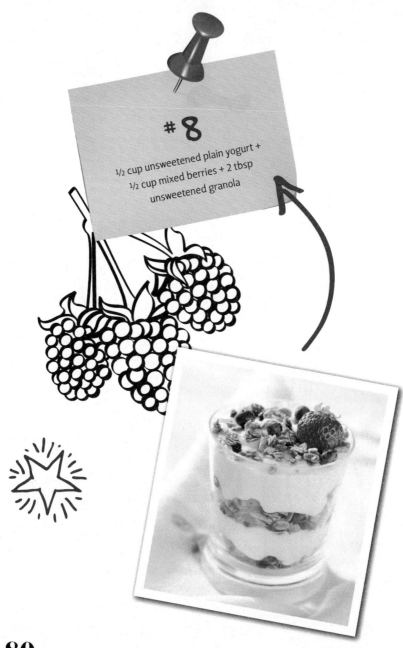

#8

½ cup unsweetened plain yogurt +
½ cup mixed berries + 2 tbsp
unsweetened granola

35

Get moving

Our bodies were made to run, jump and play. They were made to move and lately we haven't been doing a whole lot of that. It isn't hard to get up and take a walk, but most of us choose not to. We'd rather channel surf than actually get up on the board. Enough is enough. Make a pact with yourself today that you will get moving. And it doesn't have to take all day. I'm in the gym 35 to 45 minutes, five or six days each week. I lift weights, mainly, but you can choose to do whatever activity you want as long as it gets your heart pumping and body moving. Even walking to the end of the driveway is a great goal. Then tomorrow you can walk to the end of street. Or venture into the gym, grab some weights off the rack and see how good they make you feel. Movement is an incredible tool. It makes you feel good and it makes you look good. Do it now!

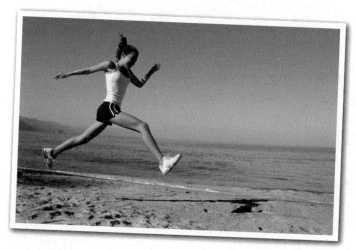

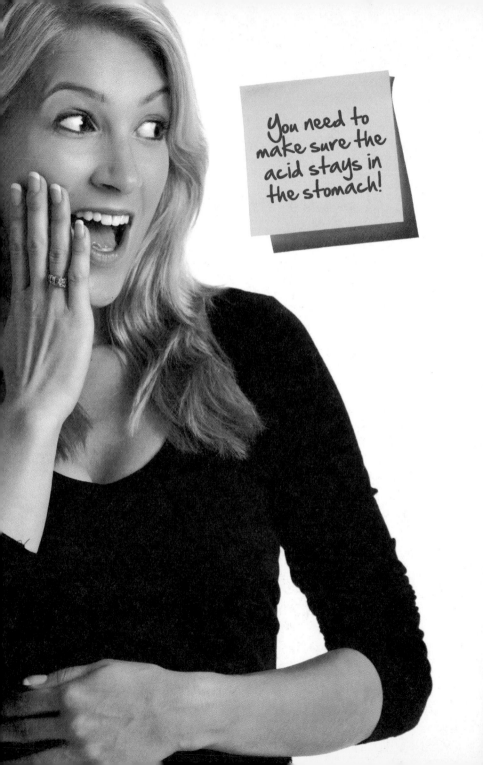

36

More acid, not less!

The trouble with digestion is you need to break your food into its little tiny bits. Acid is just the bad guy to do the job, except two-thirds of North Americans don't have enough stomach acid. Shocked? I'll bet you are, since every other ad on TV is for lowering stomach acid. Folks think that when they have heartburn or gastric reflux disease they need to kill the acid, but this is not the case. You need to make sure the acid stays in the stomach, which usually means improving your diet! (You knew I was going to say that!) Stomach acid is your first line of defense against disease, infection and a host of other problems. Let your food be your medicine and let your tummy juices do their job well. Eat Clean every day and take in a little vinegar before your meals. Yes, really! Don't like the idea of vinegar? You can take a hydrochloric acid supplement before meals instead.

Brown is best

Oats are for big and little kids

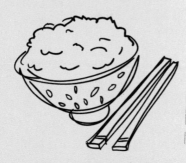

Healthy fats, healthy fun

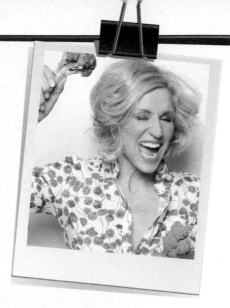

Food
Basics

37

Can you say quinoa? Or kefir?

Ever heard of these? Quinoa (pronounced keen-wah) and kefir (pronounced kuh-feer) are superfoods. These are the acceptable foods you may not have known how to pronounce as opposed to those unpronounceable ingredients mentioned in Rule #16 (pg. 40).

Why super? Well in layman's terms it's because they are superb for your health and body and they promote weight loss. Yes, healthy foods can promote weight loss. A proper definition for "superfood" refers to foods that are high in phytonutrient content and as a result provide superior health

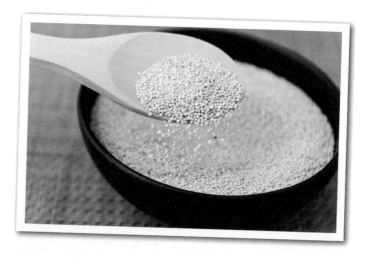

benefits. Phytonutrient is a fancy word for various health-aiding chemicals that naturally occur in plants. Contrary to chemicals in man-made foods, these chemicals actually provide nutrition and health benefits. Foods like these are fantastic for filling you up with only the best nutrition, leaving you satisfied and properly nourished. You'll be craving superfoods all the time. This is one craving I strongly recommend you feed!

Find new superfoods by researching and shopping at local markets or your organic grocer. I have recently added kombucha, enoki, adzuki and matcha to my "can't pronounce it" superfood list. Add these new foods to your diet and experience how much better you feel. You'll be surprised by what real food and proper nutrition can actually do. Your health will prove the wonders of these foods.

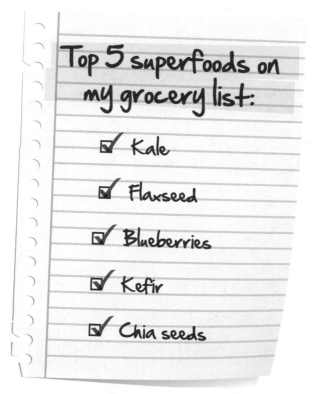

Top 5 superfoods on my grocery list:

- ☑ Kale
- ☑ Flaxseed
- ☑ Blueberries
- ☑ Kefir
- ☑ Chia seeds

38

Sugar - the legal cocaine

It's white, powdery and gives you a high – a rush of energy to accomplish anything. It's legal and it's in practically everything North Americans consume. What is it? It's sugar, an anti-food I like to call "the White Poison."

Read up on sugar and then remember what you discover, because sugar will kill you, much like its illegal doppelgänger cocaine. Sugar will leave you strung out, but also fat and injecting yourself with insulin to combat diabetes.

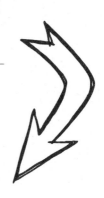

Check out some of my favorite resources on the dangers of sugar:

★ *Sugar Blues*, by William Dufty

★ *Suicide by Sugar: A Startling Look at Our #1 National Addiction*, by Nancy Appleton

★ NancyAppleton.com

★ http://www.youtube.com/watch?v=hF8XnU4L33U

★ http://www.youtube.com/watch?v=62JMfv0tf3Q

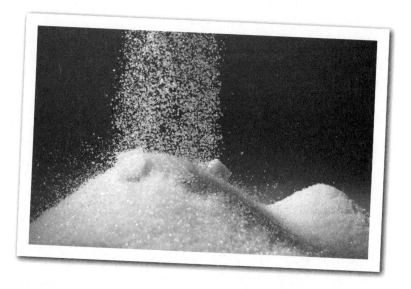

People can't leave sugar alone because they're addicted. In fact, most people today are sugar addicts – high on the sweet, delicious taste of this substance. Sugar addicts will do anything to get their fix – searching coworkers' offices for candy, scrounging for loose change to buy Coke from the vending machine, causing scenes when there is no sugar or sweetener available for their afternoon coffee. The more sugar an addict has, the more sugar he/she needs, until it spirals out of control into obesity, diabetes, chronic headaches, migraines, insomnia, ADD and ADHD, anxiety, nervousness and hosts of other health problems. Sugar should be locked up with cocaine as its cellmate, yet sugar is still legal.

Have I scared you? Good! Get sugar out of your diet today if it's the only thing you do. Don't even put it in your coffee or tea. Your taste buds will learn to live without it. In fact, once they get used to a sugar-free diet, they will reject sugar if you were to ever put it in your mouth again.

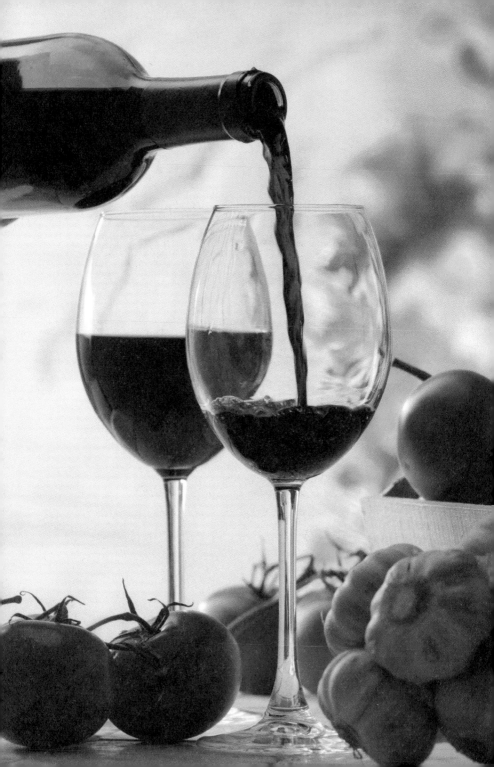

39

Alcohol – the other legal drug

Oh, alcohol! Like food it seems to be at the forefront of our social gatherings, celebrations and relaxation time. It's also one of the first things I am asked about when I host seminars: "What about alcohol?" Or "I can't live without my red wine." While alcohol such as red wine has its antioxidant benefits, it also has its share of troubles. What people seem to forget is that alcohol is a form of sugar. It's a simple form of energy that can cause you to pack on the pounds. It's also like any other drug in the sense that your liver has to work hard to process it and get it out of your system. It's easy to become addicted to it. And don't forget that drinking alcohol makes you more likely to slip up on your *Eat-Clean Diet* plan. Let's make a deal. I won't tell you to ditch alcohol altogether, but I will tell you to save it for special occasions. And before you argue about antioxidants, remember you can get them from unfermented berries, too!

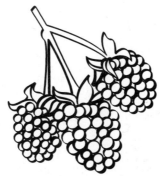

40

LP + CC sitting in a tree!

K-i-s-s-i ... well you get the point! More likely lean protein (LP) and complex carbohydrates (CC) will be sitting together on your plate or in your cooler instead. Either way, lean protein should never stray far from complex carbs and vice versa.

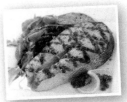

An *Eat-Clean Diet* follower knows that neither one is complete without the other when it comes to your diet and your health. In order to experience a fat-burning, metabolism-boosting energy peak you must consume both lean protein and complex carbs every two or three hours, making five or six meals per day.

So what is LP? Many options exist: chicken, turkey, salmon, white fish (in safe and healthy amounts), lean cuts of red meat, game, egg whites, beans and legumes, tofu, quinoa, sea vegetables, nuts and nut butters.

CCs are equally abundant and are found in whole grains and fresh fruit and vegetables. Foods such as oats, brown rice, quinoa, whole-grain breads and any fruits and vegetables found in your produce aisle are CCs.

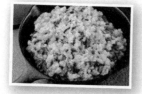

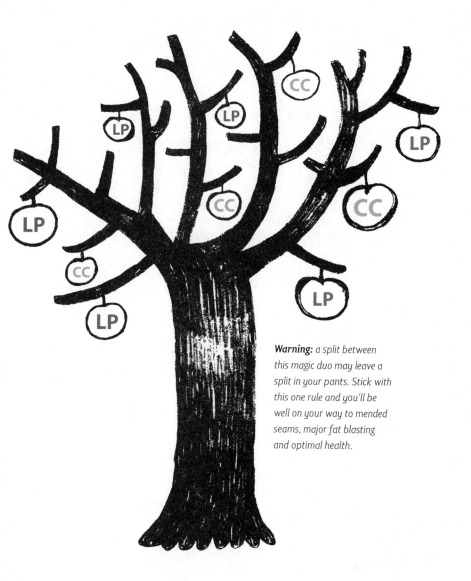

Warning: a split between this magic duo may leave a split in your pants. Stick with this one rule and you'll be well on your way to mended seams, major fat blasting and optimal health.

41

Water, water everywhere, yet some don't drink a drop!

And there is plenty to drink.

Water is everywhere! It is present in every living thing. Heck, it makes up almost 70 percent of our bodies. We need it! It's time to trade in those OJ glasses for water glasses.

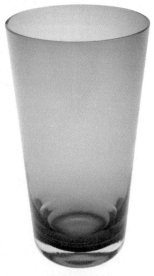
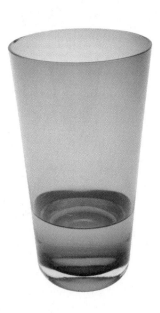
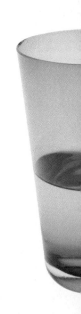

You'd never see a squirrel sipping a nice cold Coke, nor would you feed your vegetable garden a bucket of orange juice. These living creatures drink water and so should you – and you should drink a lot of it!

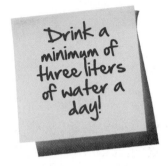

Water is used to assimilate macronutrients, vitamins and minerals, and to flush out toxins and waste. Hydration through water allows the body to perform all its functions in the most successful and efficient way. Need one more benefit? Drinking water also increases your metabolism. In addition, when you get used to drinking water you will be far less likely to take in calories through your drinks. Those juices, sodas and other sweetened drinks add up quickly!

How much should you drink? At minimum you should drink three liters of water a day. That's eight 12-ounce cups.

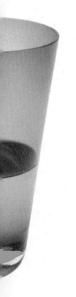
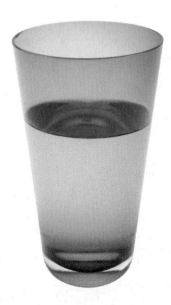
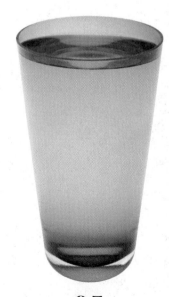

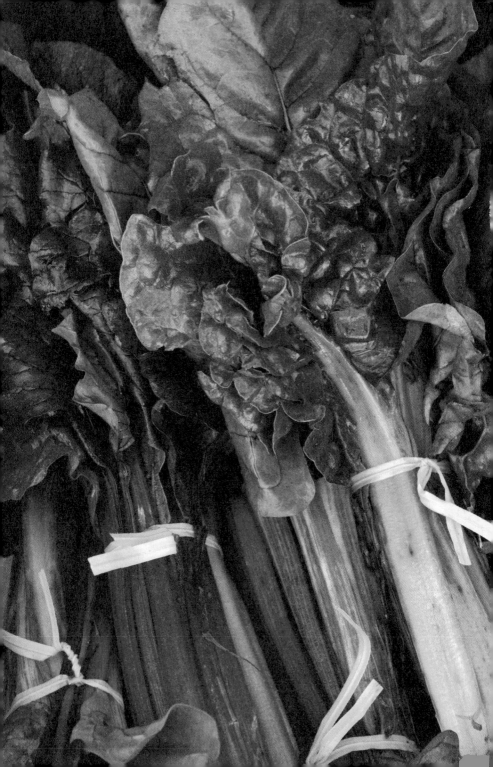

Green is not just for growing

Jump on that green bandwagon!

Consider the use of the term "growing" for more than just a garden. Greens, as I will explain in more detail, will grow you a strong and healthy body, too.

There is no doubt that greens such as broccoli, Brussels sprouts and all leafy greens (kale, spinach, collard greens and Swiss chard, for a few examples) are good for you. Greens are jam-packed with nutrients and minerals just waiting to help your body ward off disease and cancers. Greens are nutritional powerhouses rich in vitamins K, C, E and B. They are also a concentrated source of iron, calcium, potassium and magnesium.

MAJOR PLUS: These yummy leaves are low in carbohydrates and calories, so eating loads of them will not increase your waistline. If you want to see some drastic improvements in your health, eat at least six to eight cups weekly. I am so hooked on greens they end up in everything from cookies to soup.

You can eat greens with every meal: spinach in your omelets, romaine for lunch and kale with tomato sauce for dinner. Mmmmmmmm health!

43

Protein is more than just meat

Many people are under the impression that protein exists only in meat. While meat is a rich protein source, this nutrient can also be found in many other delicious food sources, which often have nutritional profiles equal to, if not greater than, meat.

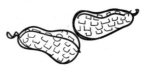

Consider eggs, fish, vegetable protein, nuts, low-fat dairy, sea vegetables and seeds. These options are leaner than meat because they are lower in saturated and trans fats and higher in fiber. Unfortunately, the protein in many plant sources is not considered complete. A complete protein contains all nine essential amino acids in proportions necessary to meet the dietary needs of a human. Thus meat alternatives such as legumes, beans, nuts and seeds need to be eaten in conjunction with specific other foods. For example, red kidney beans and brown rice make a complete protein.

Diversifying your meals with alternative forms of protein will help to freshen up your meal plans. Doing so will also introduce different nutrients into an already Clean diet. Try some of the following options when you are wondering what to snack on for protein.

 # 1 **Protein spreads:** nut and seed butters and hummus

#2 **Nuts:** almonds, cashews, peanuts, sunflower seeds, pumpkin seeds, beans and lentils

#3   **Soy products:** tempeh or tofu (tofu should be consumed in small amounts once or twice per week)

#4   **Fish:** all kinds of fish and seafood are excellent protein alternatives (watch advisories on healthy versus toxic fish types)

#5   **Eggs:** eggs are a complete protein and one of the best choices of protein for an *Eat-Clean Diet* follower. Be sure to consume more egg white than yolk; use the 3:1 ratio (3 egg whites to 1 yolk). Since I eat so many eggs I try hard to find free-range or organic eggs.

#6   **Quinoa:** I've told you how I love this stuff. Ounce for ounce quinoa contains more readily digestible and complete protein than a glass of milk. This is especially good news for vegetarians, vegans or those with dairy intolerances.

Don't forget to eat nuts, seeds, legumes and beans with whole grains such as brown rice or quinoa to obtain all the essential amino acids required by humans.

If you do opt for traditional meat sources, spice things up sometimes by opting for game meats including bison, ostrich, venison, boar or rabbit.

44

Flaxseed every day!

Nature's scrub brush

Everything feels better after a good scrub, even your intestines. Flaxseed acts like a toothbrush for your intestines and digestive system – clearing out those pipes. Eat too much and you'll be clearing out more than just that! Although it's an ancient food, flaxseed is now touted as a modern-day miracle food. I suggest it as an *Eat-Clean Diet* follower's first choice for nutrition. We know that two tablespoons of ground flaxseed every morning will help you create the healthiest body with the best digestion. A great start

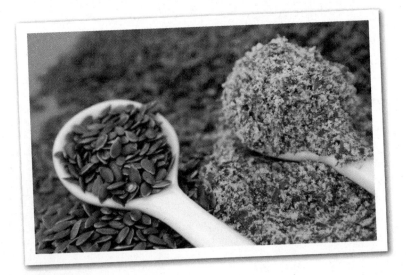

to Eating Clean is to buy some flaxseed, grind it up and start eating it! Put it on top of oatmeal, salads, yogurt, smoothies, baking – anything! I even put flaxseed into my burgers. This little seed will surprise you with its power.

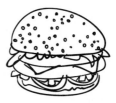

A little brown seed full of fiber and healthy oils, the flaxseed must be ground for our bodies to experience all of its goodness; otherwise it just passes right through our system whole. I recommend grinding your flaxseeds at home before using them instead of buying those already ground. Pre-ground flaxseeds lose their nutrients and go rancid more quickly.

Flaxseed offers a long list of health benefits including decreasing risk of heart disease and breast cancer and moderating many symptoms of menopause, such as those pesky hot flashes. Words of advice for the first-time user: warn your kids and spouse, and lock your bathroom door! This little seed has a serious cleansing effect! Start moderately, with just a small teaspoon, working your way up to two to four tablespoons a day.

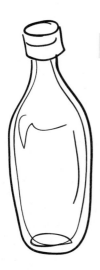

Flaxseed products:

★ **Oil:** consume a spoonful (soothes inflamed intestines)

★ **Ground:** use as a topping on most things (best for health benefits)

★ **Whole seeds:** toasted seeds can be consumed as a snack or topping, but you will not experience all of the benefits of consuming the ground seed

45

Sea salt only!

92 Versus 2

This rule is pretty straightforward: if you must eat salt, eat sea salt. Throw that table salt over your shoulder. Table salt contains two nutrients while sea salt contains ninety-two nutrients. Table salt contains any number of anti-caking agents, some of which contain aluminum. Some brands even contain sugar! (Remember the White Poison? Rule #38, pg. 88). Sea salt contains the minerals iron, sulfur and magnesium, to name a few, which help to promote efficient functioning of the liver, kidneys and adrenal glands. They also help you sleep! On the contrary, table salt will only deteriorate your health, causing high blood pressure, and heart and kidney disease. You and your savory dishes deserve only the best – so replace that table salt shaker with salt from the sea – you'll also use less salt for the same flavor.

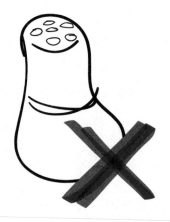

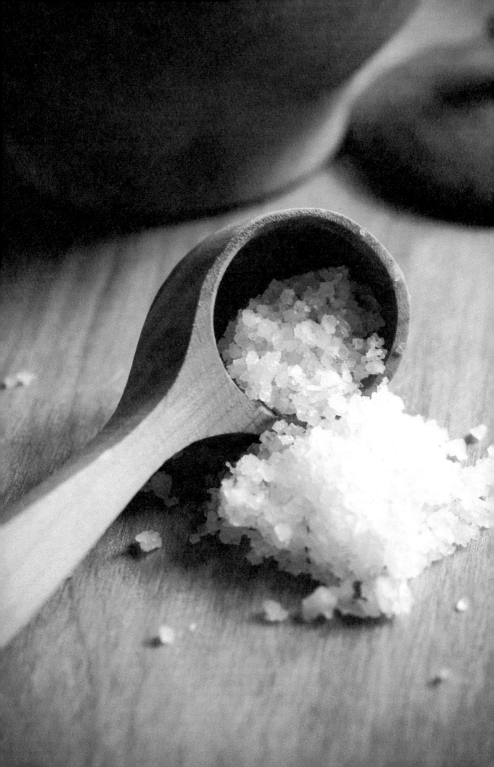

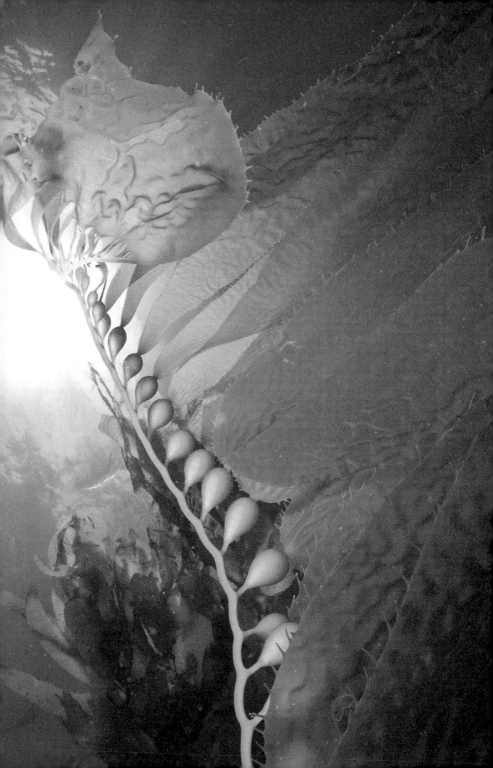

46

Sea vegetables

Eat your veggies whether they have been grown in the soil or the water. Yes water! Sea vegetables are the next greatest nutrient-rich food source coming your way and we are just getting around to realizing how great they are. Our ancestors would be laughing at us since they knew about these superfoods ages ago. Let's get up to speed and start reintroducing kelp, seaweed, wakame and more. They come in greens, reds, browns, blue-greens and more wonderful colors. Talk about nutrient rich! Sea veggies contain tons of iron, iodine, vitamins, mucilages, minerals and so much more. When I am hungry I just chomp on a sheet of nori. Yum!

47

Oats are for big and little kids

"They're mushy." "They look ugly." "Blah! Mom this tastes bad. Where's the brown sugar?" Regardless of what those little guys might say about oats, this grain should be the first thing in their (and your) mouths every day. Oats make for a perfectly nutritious breakfast and with the right toppings, a big steaming bowl of oatmeal is absolutely delicious!

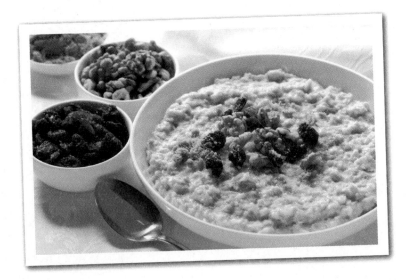

Oats are full of healthy dietary fiber, including soluble fiber. This fills your child and you, the adult, up longer than those sugar-filled cereals. This fiber helps regulate blood sugar and is known to protect against early-onset diabetes. Oats have been shown in studies to help prevent heart disease.

When your busy family is off and running it's hard to keep them well fed. Having oats for breakfast is a quick and easy way to ensure that everyone in your household has started off with the best nutrition.

Topping ideas:

★ Small amount of honey or pure maple syrup, to sweeten

★ Berries – raspberries, blueberries, strawberries, blackberries – whatever is in season!

★ Banana slices

★ Cinnamon

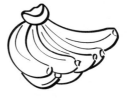

★ Dried fruit – raisins, dried cranberries, apples or apricots

★ Almond slivers

★ Seeds – pumpkin, sunflower, flax or chia

★ Bee pollen

★ Unsweetened applesauce

★ Pumpkin

48

What to put on your oats

My day is not complete without a bowl of oatmeal. I start every day off on the right foot by scooping steel-cut oats into my bowl. The next best thing is what I put on top of my oats. Wheat germ, bee pollen and flaxseed are my staples. I also add a handful of berries. Wheat germ is an excellent source of vitamin E, fiber, folic acid and antioxidants. Bee pollen is jammed full of vitamins and minerals. It's no wonder it's referred to as the perfect food. It is said that bee pollen helps with everything from energy to memory. I'm sure we could all use a boost of both! I talk about flaxseed a lot in all of my books and seminars. It's one food I sincerely would have a hard time living without. Simply add one tablespoon each of wheat germ, bee pollen and flaxseed for the perfect accompaniment to the delicious, nutritious oats you will eat every morning. Add a handful of berries on top and you've now nixed the need for brown sugar, too. It doesn't get any better than this.

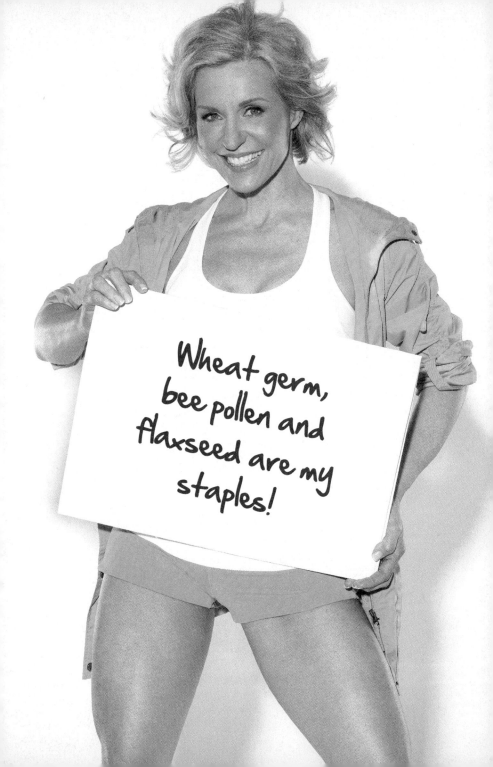

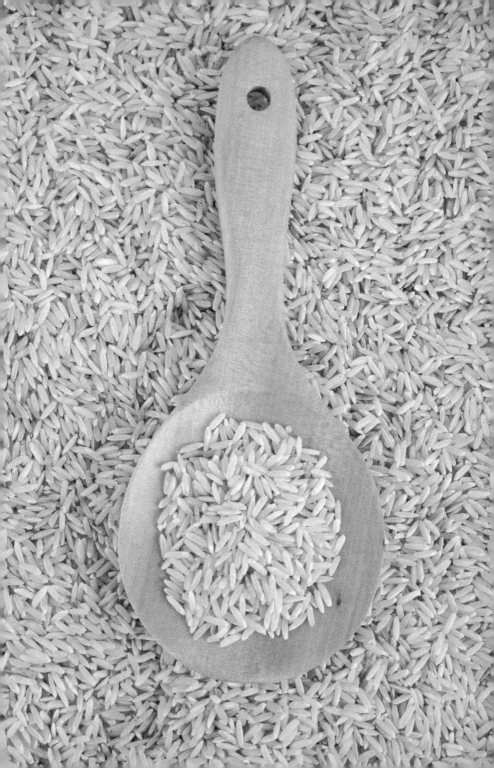

49

Brown is best

Grains and produce have come to us from nature dressed to the nines, wearing bran, germ, husk, fiber, peel and more. To eat the entire food is to gain the complete package of goodness nature intended for us. Eating only the polished white part of the rice or wheat, for example, is a mistake. Without the nutritious brown fibrous parts of these foods we are eating a lethal weapon that causes blood sugar levels to escalate. We then ask a lot of our pancreas, which has to spit out insulin to deal with the rising blood sugar. In time and with repeated insults, our cells ignore the high levels of insulin and we are no longer able to control blood sugar, leading to a state of disease called type 2 diabetes mellitus. Rice is not naturally white and isn't meant to be white if you were to ask Mother Nature. It comes in many colors from black to brown, red to pink. We have to eat all parts for optimal health.

Rice is not naturally white and isn't meant to be white if you were to ask Mother Nature.

50

Healthy fats, healthy fun

Fat runs your machine. It keeps your noggin thinking, your hormones flowing and your juices running. Don't run away from fat! Learn to lube with the right stuff. Coconut, olive, avocado, flaxseed and pumpkin seed oils are some of my current favorites. I feel their love on salads and in my cooking, and I even use coconut oil to moisturize my hair and skin! Good fats like these are sure to keep you lean since they also stoke your metabolic rate and that means fuel-burning consumption running on high. Start with two tablespoons a day and say "How *you* doin'?!"

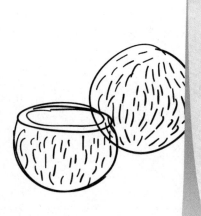

I even use coconut oil to moisturize my hair and skin!

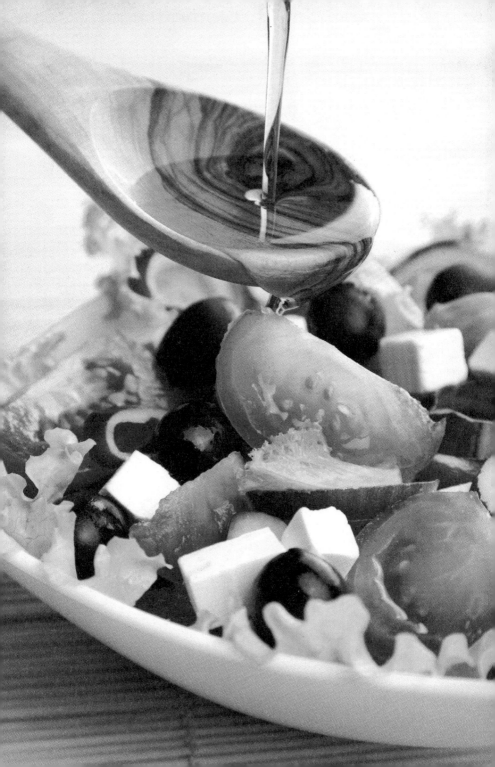

51

Food, not pills

If you Eat Clean you will be much less likely to pop countless amounts of pills, whether nutritional or pharmaceutical. Eating Clean brings you to another nutritional level altogether, where the quality ingredients your body needs to run optimally come from food rather than a pill. Imagine that! All we need to survive is packed into delicious food sources rather than plastic bottles. Better yet, with a healthy dietary regimen you are much less likely to put yourself in a state of poor health where pharmaceutical drugs are required. Surprise! You can put your pennies back in your piggy bank and load up on Eat-Clean food for your optimal health.

Please do keep in mind that there are always situations in which our bodies need a little extra help, such as when we encounter uncontrollable health and environmental conditions. For example, the current state of our food's growing conditions is troubled thanks to depleted soils from overfarming, excessive use of fertilizers, herbicides and pesticides and polluted waters. This results in fewer minerals and vitamins in our foods and makes an argument for nutritional supplements. There are also loads of folks who don't have access to information about nutrition, and there are

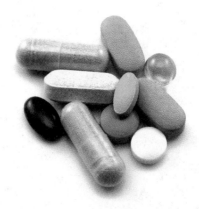

others still who live in compromised conditions where access to good food is impossible. In these cases a good-quality multivitamin could help give them what they are lacking. Work with your healthcare professional to be sure you are on the right track and are not in need of any of the following, which are the most commonly lacking vitamins, minerals and nutraceuticals:

★ Vitamin D because of a lack of healthy sun exposure. In some northern countries rickets is making a comeback thanks to insufficient sun and too much sunblock!

★ Fish oil in health-maintaining or therapeutic doses. Eating enough fish oil may help keep your mood in top form. Some mental health practitioners are using therapeutic doses of fish oil to fight depression, inflammation, heart disease and macular degeneration.

★ Vitamin K for fighting rickets.

★ Calcium along with weight-bearing exercise for strong bones and teeth.

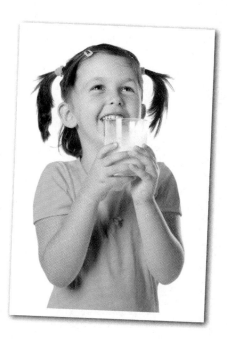

★ HCL (hydrochloric acid) to optimize stomach acid contents for seamless digestion. Without it you can eat as Clean and wholesome as you like and not gain any benefit. Most North Americans do not have enough!

★ Adrenal support to address a nationwide epidemic of chronic stress and disease. A few drops will put you back in the nutritional driver's seat.

Eating Clean is simple

Kick out the crap

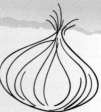

It's never too late to start!

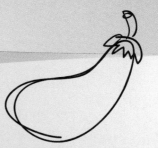

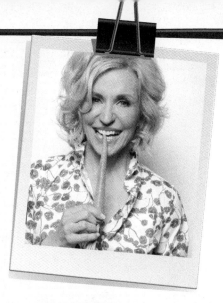

Last
Words

Last Words on Eating Clean

This isn't a complicated message. In fact, Eating Clean is as simple as it can get. So what's the bottom line? Eat a wide variety of wholesome, natural foods by combining lean protein with complex carbohydrates from fruits, vegetables and whole grains. Kick out the crap, invite in the good, throw in some water and you are on your way to excellent health and a better body than you've ever imagined. Is this information new? No. It's the same information we've heard from our ancestors time and time again. The difference is the package. *Just the Rules* puts it all into perspective in a handy pocket guide that tells you when it's time to put down the chips and pick up the carrots. Why? Because without this way of eating you will wind up overweight, sick and tired. Why else? Because you can, and it's never too late to start!

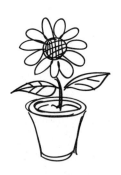

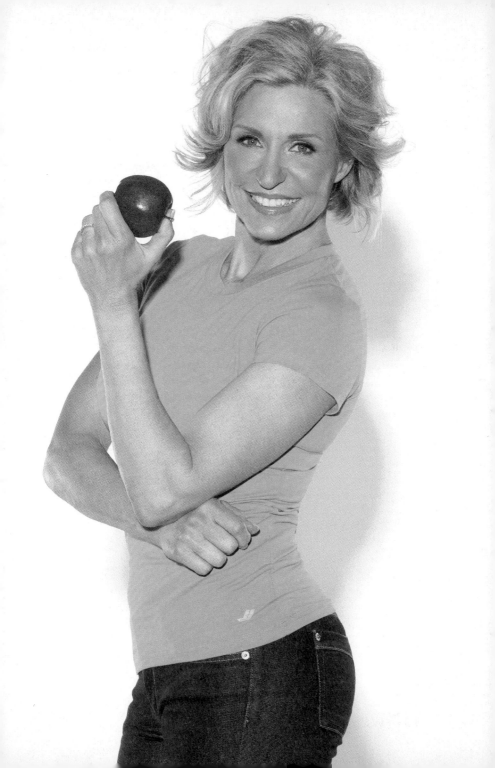

Acknowledgments

Sometimes in life the rules are meant to be broken, but when it comes to nourishing your body, don't mess with the rules.

Here are my thanks to the people whose rules I follow so that I can share mine with you:

Thanks to my husband, Robert Kennedy, for introducing me to the rules of the road and the tricks of the trade for Eating Clean. You gave me the foundation I needed to create a plan that speaks to so many people in so many different ways. And I hope to reach even more people with this simple, quick read. Thank you.

A very special thank you goes out to my daughter, Kiersten. Her spicy character and special way with words shaped and inspired this latest book. She's a no-nonsense girl and she needed a no-nonsense plan. Kiersten, my talented social media queen, this book is for you! Thanks for all that you do to keep me in the present. Readers can connect with Kiersten on The Kitchen Table, your online support system, at eatcleandiet.com/the_kitchen_table

As usual, I need to say a special thank you to the Robert Kennedy Publishing Book Department for their hours and hours of labor on this project. Who knew that a book so small could take up so much time? From ironing out the best rules to share with you, to filming fun videos, to editing, designing and more, *Just the Rules* was a team project just like every other book in the *Eat-Clean Diet*® series.

In particular...

Big, warm hugs of acknowledgment go directly to Wendy Morley and Gabriella Caruso Marques. These two wonder women are the reason my books sound and look as good as they do. To Wendy Morley for keeping me in line both on the page and in my work, and to Gabby for creating beautiful images out of my written words.

Thanks also to Amy Land for her editing prowess, to Brittany Seki for being me when I can't be, to Meredith Barrett for keeping me online, to Christopher Barnes for creating my sites, to Sharlene Liladhar for organizing me, to Patricia D'Amato for knowing my market, to Kelsey-Lynn Corradetti and Chelsea Kennedy for your assistance whenever it is needed, for food and fashion at our many photo shoots (and for also being wonderfully supportive children), to Brian Ross, Jessica Pensabene and Ellie Jeon for their book design skills and support for Gabby, and to Rachel Corradetti for her additions sprinkled throughout the book and for also being another supportive daughter milling about the office.

Last but certainly not least...

A special thank you to my many coworkers who have been with me since the early stages of *The Eat-Clean Diet®* series. We've grown and developed into a strong and thriving information hub, fostering healthy change in the lives of men and women of all ages. But as we grow bigger, we still maintain our roots. Many of the roots are the work of Vinita Persaud, who is now moving on to bigger and better things. Thanks for all of your knowledge over the years. You'll be missed.

And finally...

To you! My reader. You are the most important part of this equation because you had the motivation to pick up this book. You have made a small choice that will set you on the right path to creating your best self. Congratulations! Are you ready to follow the rules?

Goals

Setting goals is the key to success. Each goal is a stepping stone toward your ideal self. Give yourself reasonable goals to work toward. Rather than trying to lose 20 pounds in one week, strive for 2 pounds. You can try for 20 pounds over time.

Breaking your long-term goal down into attainable short-term goals keeps you aware of your progress, and you are constantly rewarding yourself by completing one step toward a better you!

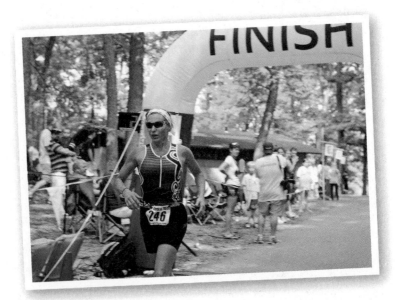

Weekly Goals

Making positive changes each week will add up. You'll start seeing results in no time!

By this time next week...

_____
_____
_____

Monthly Goals

Some of your goals will take a little longer. Choose a few monthly goals and stick to the changes you've already made.

By this time next month...

_____
_____
_____

Long-Term Goals

Studies have shown that people who write down their long-term goals are more successful in many aspects of life than those who do not. Do it now!

By this time next year...

_____
_____
_____

Weekly Goals

Making positive changes each week will add up. You'll start seeing results in no time!

By this time next week...

_____

_____

_____

Monthly Goals

Some of your goals will take a little longer. Choose a few monthly goals and stick to the changes you've already made.

By this time next month...

_____

_____

_____

Long-Term Goals

Studies have shown that people who write down their long-term goals are more successful in many aspects of life than those who do not. Do it now!

By this time next year...

_____

_____

_____

Weekly Goals

Making positive changes each week will add up. You'll start seeing results in no time!

By this time next week...

_____

_____

_____

Monthly Goals

Some of your goals will take a little longer. Choose a few monthly goals and stick to the changes you've already made.

By this time next month...

_____

_____

_____

Long-Term Goals

Studies have shown that people who write down their long-term goals are more successful in many aspects of life than those who do not. Do it now!

By this time next year...

_____

_____

_____

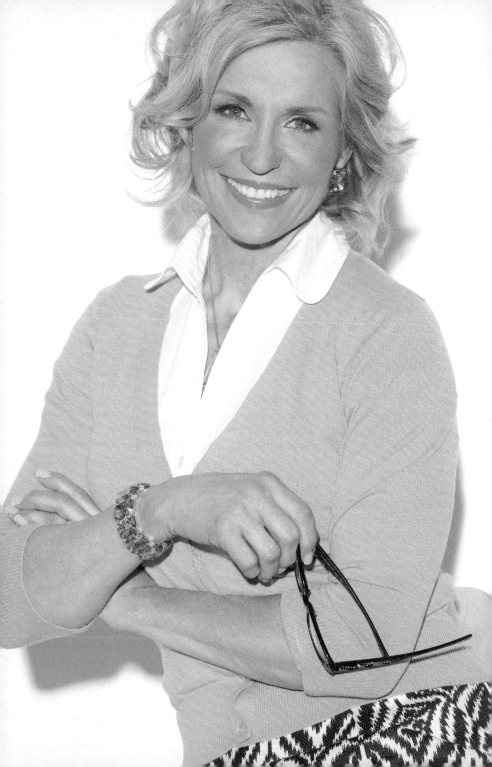